COMFORTABLE PAIN

The inspirational story of a nurse
living with multiple chronic illnesses

Dani Lee

Wishing you hope, joy + love

XO.

Leisa Cadotte

Published by Leisa Cadotte, May, 2018
ISBN: 9781775349501

Editor: Danielle Anderson
Typeset: Greg Salisbury
Book Cover Design: Judith Mazari
Portrait Photographer: Wendy Lees, Wendy Lees Ciao Bella
        Photography

DISCLAIMER: The information provided in this book is designed to provide helpful information on the subjects discussed. This book is not meant to be used, nor should it be used, to diagnose or treat any medical condition. For diagnosis or treatment of any medical problem, consult your own physician. The publisher and author are not responsible for any specific health or allergy needs that may require medical supervision and are not liable for any damages or negative consequences from any treatment, action, application or preparation, to any person reading or following the information in this book. References are provided for informational purposes only and do not constitute endorsement of any websites or other sources. Readers should be aware that the websites listed in this book may change.

Dedication

Pour François, Mathieu, et Benjamin,
Je t'aime.

Testimonials

"Leisa's story of managing multiple chronic diseases is one of a kind. Not only does she combine her experiences and hardships but, she also addresses an admirable and firm faith in God by trusting His purpose for her life, even when faced with circumstances that would dishearten most. As her doctor, to see her approach the ups and downs of her illness with perseverance while always looking for the good in difficult situations is completely inspirational."
Dr. Evaristus Idanwekhai, MBBS, CCFP, Chief Medical Director and founder of the 1st Canadian Medical Centre

"I've had the pleasure of knowing Leisa for 10 years. I was her nursing instructor 10 years ago and worked alongside of her 6 years ago. She is the strongest person that I have ever known. She always sees the positive side to life even with all the difficulties that she has encountered over the years. She gets down sometimes but always picks herself up over and over again. I had her speak to my nursing students in their 1st semester of class and they still speak about how wonderful Leisa was. "
Anne Hamilton, RN, Nursing Instructor CDI College

"Leisa Cadotte is an inspiration unwavering courage through her toughest times of physical pain and the emotional challenges she has faced coming to terms with having to reimagine how her life would look in light of her chronic illnesses. In true Leisa style, she has found a way to continue her role as a dedicated caregiver, nurturer, and teacher. With this book, Leisa has created a legacy that offers much needed support and guidance for people navigating the healthcare

system for them or a family member. Her honest account of her experiences as a nurse and patient gives readers the knowledge and tools they need to find their best path to wellness. Leisa is a true warrior!"

Karen Pledger, Restorative Yoga Instructor

"Leisa is one of the more adventurous and bold women I know, strongly opinionated too but always with a good laugh. Without the physical challenges, who know what Leisa would have accomplished in terms of visible work and visible impact? But she was called to something more private and less visible where she had to consolidate all the energies of her bold heart and the stamina of her adventurous spirit to tackle the personal challenges she has had to face.

Some might value the visible over the invisible, In fact many do and as a result those burdened by personal sickness can easily bemoan their situation and live their days consumed with disappointment, sadness, bitterness and anger. It is a different sort of adventure to struggle with the invisible and painful realities of a malfunctioning body and to remain alive to the opportunities to live fully in the world. It demands the development of a deep hope. It calls for great resources beyond the earthly. It compels great humility as one depends on the strengths of the one above and the strengths of those around.

Leisa shares how her faith in Christ guided her through the turmoil of sickness, uncertain diagnosis, and experimental medications. Her reflections on this journey are shaped by a growing and developing Christian faith that intersects with her background in emergency response and nursing. For those struggling with chronic sickness, Leisa invites you to share in her story and to learn from that story.

I encourage you to read this book as though Leisa was sitting beside you. She gets what you are struggling with. As she tells her stories, pick up that she is also telling the story of how God seeks to journey with you as He did with her. The more you make room for God to work in your life, the more you will be filled with a new hope and a new energy that turns the tide against disappointment and sadness. You will begin to find that God has a particular purpose even in your sickness. Much of your personal struggle may be invisible to most people, but the visible outcomes of your invisible struggles, if well engaged, will become a blessing and an encouragement to many.

Besides, when was the last time you heard a well-experienced nurse who needs the expert care of nurses and doctors, tell it like it really is. Enjoy this read which combines the advances of science and the mysteries of the spiritual. You will be blessed."

Executive Pastor Jim Heuving, Pacific Community Church

"This book may seem like a small light in the blackest night of pervasive sickness in our society. But it's a bright light for many who are struggling with health challenges. This book, I think, provides a beacon of light and hope for many who struggle with chronic illness. You will learn that if one individual, with a determined mindset, can manage to make it through multiple chronic health illnesses, then certainly, you can do it too."

Dr. C. Leong Wong, DC, FCCPOR(C), DACRB, CCC

"Leisa's wealth of knowledge, contagious laugh and terrible attempt at accents, let you know she is someone that will make a huge impact on people's lives in the most positive way. As a close friend and colleague, never did she ever display any sign of an internal struggle. It wasn't until a couple of years ago, did she share her story of the chronic challenges she had to fight with every day. I was in complete shock as Leisa had to occupy herself with the many roles she played. This gave me immeasurable respect for her and motivated me to gain more insight on the scale and impact that chronic conditions have on people's lives and families. Leisa is a reminder of what a survivor is. This book is a paradigm highlighting the importance of awareness that is needed to draw attention to the spectrum of chronic illnesses. I am honored to have met Leisa, fortunate to have worked at her side, and blessed to call her my friend."

Hadiah Mizban, LPN, HCA Instructor

Acknowledgements

Thank you to the amazing Julie Salisbury, my friend and publisher of Influence Publishing, for your dedication to your craft and your gentle but firm hand, which kept me from the edge of quitting while I was writing. Thank you also to the talented Wendy Lees and her gift of not only the amazing photographs for the covers of the book, but for her encouragement as well. Danielle Anderson, thank you for your skilled editor's insight on how to pull this entire book together. I would like to acknowledge my doctor's, specialists, and surgeons for listening to me and treating me with respect. Thank you to Barb Wallick and Teri Holland for coaching me to stay focused on my positive beliefs and overcoming my fears.

Where would I be without my friends and family? Thanks for sticking by me not just during the creation of the book, but for being there when it counted the most—while I was ill or in pain. Thank you to our friends, who have loved me both when I'm well and when I'm not and including me either way. You know who you are. My journey has been blessed with amazing parents— Sherran, Tom, and Lisa. Without your support and unconditional love, this book would not have been possible. Thank you to my loving sister Andi, whom amazes me and inspires me in so many ways. Thank you for the love and support from our family in Montreal, and for our sons Mathieu and Benjamin, who remind me of my everyday purpose in life. A special *merci* to my husband François for stepping up and the running of the household when I couldn't, for pushing me forward when I needed a kick in the butt, and especially for holding me back when rest was essential for our survival. If not for his love, this book would never have been written. Praise God for His strength, patience, protection and the hand that guides my path.

Contents

Synopsis

After twenty exciting years in Emergency and Health Care Services, Leisa retires due to her own serious health complications. Her experience in Disaster Response, Search & Rescue, Surgical Nursing and finally as a Health Care Educator gives her the expertise she would need to become her own patient advocate.

This inspiring author survives a stroke at age thirty-five, is diagnosed with multiple life-threatening illness, and is given a not-so-promising outlook for what the future would hold for her and her family. This allows her to discover her own inner strength and find a strong hope for a better life.

Leisa's uplifting story takes us on a journey of how she navigates our complicated healthcare system while coping with debilitating chronic pain. Through her humorous accounts of the challenges she faces as both the nurse and the patient, the author teaches us how love, faith, and laughter are the best medicine.

"Character cannot be developed in ease and quiet. Only through experience of trial and suffering can the soul be strengthened, ambition inspired, and success achieved."
Hellen Keller

Foreword

When I first met Leisa I knew she was a gift, sent to me so I could learn more about my own battle with chronic pain.

I am constantly inspired by Leisa's determination and courage, and by how she honours her body's needs. Her incredible journey has inspired me to treat my own body with more care and respect, and to share my pain with my family so they can help me live within my limitations. Many times, I have fallen into the trap of "suffering in silence" so as not to be a burden on my loved one or pushing myself to do activities that will cause me pain because I feel like I *should* be able to do them. By sharing her personal experience of learning to live with multiple chronic illnesses, Leisa showed me that those who truly care about you want you to be honest about how you feel so that you don't have to experience more pain.

Leisa has also taught me that as someone living with an invisible illness, it is up to me to ask for help. When you aren't obviously ill, people will not automatically step in and offer assistance when you need it. Her lessons in self-care have empowered me to ask for a seat on the bus or to get someone to open the window or a heavy door for me. If I don't speak up, how can anyone know that I need help?

Leisa uses her unique perspective as a person living with multiple chronic illnesses along with her experience as a Nurse and Health Care Educator to help you learn how to manage chronic illnesses and pain, or how to care for someone suffering from these types of conditions. She explores every aspect of self-care and disease management, including topics such as alternative healing, faith and divine intervention, and mental health. She freely shares the many facets of her experience, from amusing anecdotes to heart-wrenching losses, so that those on the same path know they are not alone. She teaches you not just to survive, but to thrive. The result is a wonderful resource that gives us a better understanding of how to live with chronic illness and pain.

I am full of admiration of Leisa, and I am very grateful to be on this journey to share this wealth of information with you. I hope that this book helps your own experience with chronic pain or illnesses become a more comfortable one!

Julie Salisbury, Founder Influence Publishing Inc.

Introduction

How do you get up every day? Do you hop up out of bed, jump into the shower, hurry back to get dressed, and run downstairs to make breakfast? Do you have to plan how you're going to navigate your morning routine, or does it just happen automatically? I used to be able to quickly and easily accomplish all these simple daily tasks. I prided myself that I was never high maintenance; instead, I was an on-the-go kind of girl.

I can no longer hop, jump, hurry, or run, especially not all on the same day. That's a fact I've been facing for the past thirteen years and will continue to fight for the rest of my life, unless they find a cure for all nine or ten of my chronic illnesses.

My name is Leisa. I'm a recently-retired Nurse as well as an Instructor and Health Care Educator. Included in those titles is mother, wife, sister, daughter, and friend to many. I am also a patient living with multiple chronic illnesses, the main one being systemic lupus. Over the course of my life I have experienced a stroke, numerous kidney infections, a rare and hard-to-pronounce lung disease, high blood pressure, enlarged heart, liver problems, skin deformities, degenerative spinal discs and hip joints, daily widespread pain, and progressively fading eyesight. While this list may make my situation sound uniquely challenging, in truth there are many people out there who, like me, have to find a way to live while combating multiple health issues.

In many cases, you wouldn't know we are sick just by looking at us. Most chronic illnesses are invisible, which allows us to appear normal from the outside. When we feel good, we participate, and those are the times you see us at our so-called best. I'll let you in on a little secret though: trying to appear normal is much harder than actually fighting the illnesses. We face a never-ending battle every waking hour of each and every day. Many of us do our best to hide it, even when we are right smack in the middle of a flare-up, because we refuse to be defined by our illness. So, how does one recognize a person living with multiple serious chronic illnesses? Often you don't, unless they choose to tell you.

A few friends suggested I write a book about my experience overcoming the challenges I faced as a nurse and working mom while dealing with multiple chronic illnesses. Unsure if this is a direction I should go in, I asked God for some kind of sign that writing a book was the right thing to do at this point in my life. My first answer came in the form of encouragement from others, who were inspired upon hearing me share my story of overcoming incredible obstacles. If this path would allow me to make a difference in at least one life, then it was a path worth taking.

Within a few weeks of making this decision, an educational publishing company approached me to do a peer review on a text book that other medical professionals had written. They'd somehow tracked me down through the college I was teaching at, and they said I came highly recommended as an expert in my field. I had to read the email at least three times and double check the voicemail to make sure they had the right person. Once I received the hard copy of the text book and saw my name in print, the idea of telling my story in the form of a book became more and more exciting!

Weeks later, while attending a gala dinner fundraiser for lupus, I was inspired by one of the speakers—the adult child of a mother with lupus. As she bravely shared her story and how her parent's illness had affected her, I pictured my own children and how this disease has robbed them of part of their childhood. I could make a difference and help others with my own story of living with lupus while raising my kids and how my health challenges have shaped them into the compassionate souls they are today. Three days later came the "Aha!" moment, and I put all the signs together. I'm thinking of writing a book, a popular publishing company has sought me out to assist with the review and editing of a medical textbook, and people keep telling me I should share my story. Was it fate, destiny, coincidence, or divine intervention? Whatever it is, I'm running with it! It was only a few months later that a friend invited me to attend a women's conference, where I met my publisher, and the rest is history.

This book is focused on the past ten years of my life, which involved juggling work, parenting, marriage, and other important relationships all while struggling with diagnostic tests, debilitating symptoms from multiple chronic illnesses, depression, and the oh-so-not-wonderful side effects from a multitude of medications. I've added in a few of my personal stories taken from a journal that I have been writing in for the past few years, along with my own working knowledge as a former Nurse and Nursing Instructor in Health Care Education. At the end of each chapter, I've left a question for you, the reader, in order to keep the conversation going about invisible chronic illness, pain, and how it tests our strength and builds our courage.

The idea for this book was to take a leap of faith and, by sharing my personal experiences, deliver the message of not letting your illness control your life and about finding a sense of humour in all the craziness that comes with chronic pain. My hope is to inspire others living with chronic illness or facing challenges in their everyday lives to keep moving forward to a better you.

My wish for you is that you may find strength within yourself by using the gifts you already have or by searching for something you may be missing. Use your spirituality, faith, family, friends and medical care team; be able to ask for help, and then trust the healing process. And, most importantly, never give up!

"Success consists of going from failure to failure without loss of enthusiasm."
Unknown

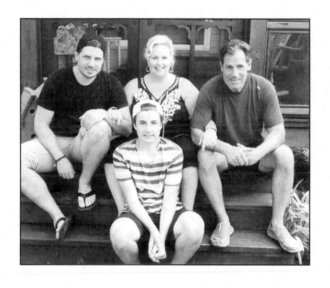

Chapter 1

How did I get here?

In order for you to understand what my chronic illnesses have taken from me and the process of my grief—the intensity of my triumphs and losses—I want to give you a glimpse of what my life was like, and what I was like, before I got sick.

I was born in the summer of 1969 beautiful British Columbia, Canada. I was the third child born but only the second to survive, following the death of my brother. He passed away on October 31, 1967, having lived only twenty-one days. Ever since, my mom has not been herself at this time of year.

Not much was said about my brother until I got older and started asking questions. I never understood why my parents didn't want to talk about his death until I became a parent myself; I can't imagine the pain they must have suffered. From the small bits of information I was given, I believe that he may have suffered some kind of autoimmune deficiency. I didn't make the connection between his condition and my own health issues until 2009—was there possibly a genetic autoimmune impairment in the family history?

Many health issues cropped up when I was growing up, but no one seemed to find them overly concerning or check if they might be interrelated. At three or four years of age I had badly infected tonsils that affected my hearing temporarily. I eventually had the tonsils removed and spent Halloween in the hospital, much to the despair of my parents; apparently I didn't care about my recovering throat, I was going to have candy even if it hurt! Eczema flare ups covered my hands, feet, and face from early childhood right up until I was a young adult. I remember having constant mouth ulcers, and still do to this day. I started having back pain in my early teens, which we chalked it up to growing pains and playing too hard in my all my sports. We would learn later that I had mild scoliosis, which was followed by osteoarthritis joint pain, three or four bulging discs in my spine, and degenerative vertebrae in my neck. In my late twenties, after a biopsy and exploratory surgery, I was diagnosed with endometriosis, which they would later perhaps incorrectly blame for the miscarriages I would have. My joints were also constantly sore when I was a teenager, but this was attributed to the fact that I played sports. Looking back, I now question when my lupus actually started to appear. I grew up in the 70's and 80's, when many doctors would have never heard of lupus. How long had I actually had this condition before I was officially diagnosed in 2005? If I had known this condition existed back then, would I have been able to recognize the symptoms? Or, would the life of athletic injuries cover it up?

Growing up in my family was a wonderful combination of structure and silliness. Both parents were fairly strict, but the household rules were ones of respect and consideration of others. As a result, my desire to care for others came at an early age.

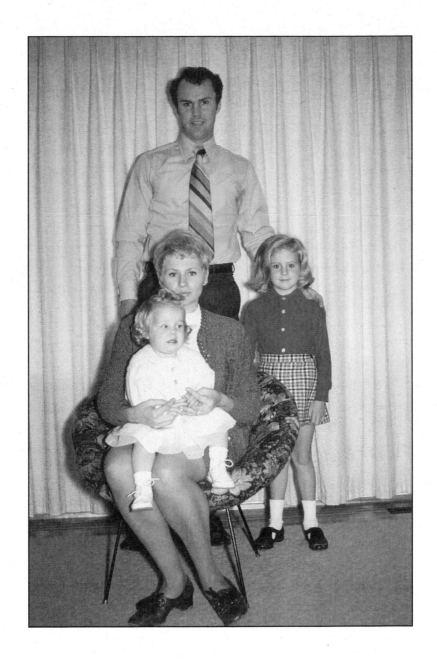

My first experience with families living with challenges came from a summer sport camp in Port Coquitlam, where I met my first mentor with a disability: Terry Fox. It was the summer of 1976, and I was seven years old. I still have the certificate with his signature on it. My kids are so amazed that I have this, and when my youngest was participating for the Terry Fox run at elementary school, he was very proud to announce to his teacher and friends that his mother had actually met him.

At this summer sport camp, I remember meeting a lot of children who didn't look like me. Some made strange noises or had unusual faces, while others drooled and screamed unidentifiable words. I can still see this large boy who looked like he was already a fully-grown man. He was standing at the top of the slide yelling "bee-bang" over and over. My seven-year-old brain thought this was confusing. What was he trying to say? Did he need help, or was he just saying hello? Was this a secret language that I didn't know about? More pressingly, though, I was concerned about his safety. He could have fallen off the top of the slide! My older sister had done that on that very same slide and broken her arm, so I was very worried for him.

I don't recall how they managed to get him down from there, but from that day forward I have had instant compassion for people with disabilities—including their struggle with communication and their right to participate in all activities.

Fast forward to my teenage years, where I became one of the very first students in the history of my high school to participate in a pilot project. We were a class of senior students assisting kids with special needs for actual course credit. It was my first real teaching experience. My tasks were different every day, but I worked mostly with kids with behavioral issues and with visual and learning disabilities. I remember it being uncool to be associated with the "awks" (short for being awkward, their words not mine) at the end of the hall; this was 1986, so political correctness was still not a thing and teenagers could be mean. I came out unscathed but determined that I would make a difference in the world. Unexpectedly, I received the prestigious service pin at graduation, reserved for only one student. This was my destiny! Helping others would be my calling!

I was a typical kid who loved sports, and I played them all. In 1977, I made my debut as a goalie on the local soccer team. By age eleven, I was the all-star pitcher for an elite fastball team. By the time I reached my teens I was ranked one of the top soccer goalies in the lower mainland on an undefeated team, played multiple positions at provincial championship-level fastball, was captain of my high school volleyball team, and recreationally competed in basketball and badminton. Do I forever hold onto these as my big achievements in life? Certainly not, (okay, maybe just a little) but they demonstrate the level of competitiveness, need for constant drive, and unswayable determination that I've had since I was a child.

Playing this hard did have its downfalls. I had reconstructive surgery on my nose from being kicked in the face while playing rugby. I suffered a few minor blackouts from hitting my head on the goal post. I had my first knee surgery at the age of sixteen, which at the time I wore as a badge of honour. I also received six stiches for getting a rock stuck in my knee. To this day some think it happened during a formidable game, but I actually tripped in the parking lot after team pictures!

As I moved into my twenties, I began pursuing my dream of attaining a post-secondary education that would lead me to my future of helping people. I wanted to live a life of service, and at the time I thought this meant going into either Law Enforcement or Therapeutic Recreation.

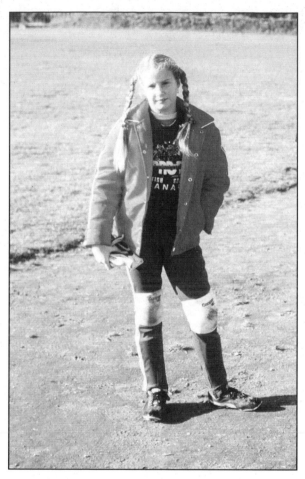

I decided to pursue a career in Law Enforcement while working at Simon Fraser University in the Continuing Studies Department. I had previous been the receptionist for the Dean's office and had assisted with the Prison Education Program, which I found very interesting! So, I enrolled at Douglas College in New Westminster, BC and started working towards obtaining my Bachelor's degree in Social Sciences.

During college, I worked part-time at a gym in White Rock, BC helping with manning the front desk, registering new members, and inspecting/cleaning/maintaining the equipment. This was my introduction into the health and fitness world. I started training at the gym, running, and earning a few belt levels in Shotokan Karate to prepare to apply with the Vancouver Police Department. There were not many females with the same goals as me, so I spent quite a bit of time with training with my male friends and completing requirements for law enforcement. I was on my way to living my dream of becoming a police officer!

Eventually I went for my physical testing, which I completed and passed flying colours. I even beat some of the guys during the physical challenges. That was awesome!

Around this time, I also volunteered with the "Crime Watch-Citizen Patrol" run by the local RCMP. I went on to complete Speed Radar training and volunteer with the BC Summer Games security team. While I had decided to pursue Law Enforcement, I decided that Therapeutic Recreation would always be in my life, even if it was only as a volunteer.

During my training in 1991, I met my husband François while he was on a seven-day work trip to Vancouver; he was a bodyguard for Prime Minister Mulroney. After a long-distance relationship, he convinced me to move to Ottawa in 1992. He flew out to meet me in BC, we packed my clothes and guitar, and then we drove my jeep across Canada to start our new life together in Quebec.

I inherited a wonderful new step-son, Mathieu, who was four-and-a-half at the time. He spoke only Quebecois, Canada's other official language, while I only spoke English. While my husband worked in Ottawa, we lived in a nearby city in Quebec.

Many of our neighbours also did not speak English, so with help from Mathieu I learned this new language very quickly—although not without a few funny miscommunications along the way!

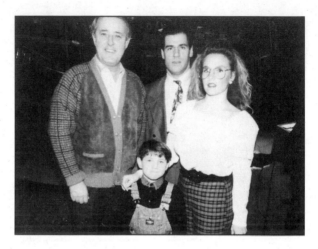

For example, the two of us were on a walk near a river, me on foot and him on his tricycle, when I tried to say to "atan," which means to wait. Instead, I got confused and said "avant," which means to go! Thankfully I managed to catch him before he got to the water's edge, but all the bystanders in the park must have thought I was insane for telling him to ride forward into the river! It was scary then, but oh how we all laugh at this story now!

While this was a very exciting and adventurous time, it was also very stressful to make such a big change in my life. We didn't know it at the time, but eventually that stress would take its toll and my health would start to go south. While nowadays stress is more commonly recognized as a connection to ill-health, at the time the theory was still relatively unknown.

For the first few months after I arrived, I worked at the

Lone Star Bar & Grill as a server to help pay with the bills. Next, I found work as a bilingual temp for an administrative pool in the Government. I worked in a few different departments including Foreign Affairs, Import and Export Sector, Revenue Canada, Air Navigation, and the Canadian Radio and Television Telecommunications (CRTC). The money was good, but I felt bored and unfulfilled. I needed to be working with my passion; I needed to be helping people. So, I volunteered at a community centre with a city-run day program for adults with disabilities. I worked with individuals with behavior problems, schizophrenia, Down syndrome, epilepsy, and traumatic brain injury along with men, women, and teens with visual and auditory impairments.

I was still hoping to get into law enforcement. My memory isn't what it used to be, so I may not have everything in chronological order, but I do remember working at Carleton University with the Campus Police Department for a few years. I started as the Administrative Assistant to the Director of what was then called Campus Security. After a while, my administrative position was on the table with the union and I was bumped out by someone with higher seniority. This was my opportunity to give the uniform one last try.

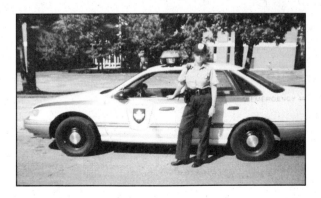

Because of my previous experience and training in Law Enforcement, along with my recent experience with the Campus Police department, going into uniform as one of the new Campus Police officers was a natural transition. Sadly, this experience would be overshadowed by a few disgruntled officers who, unaware of my previous background, misunderstood my transition from the Directors office as being favouritism. I was subjected to some unfortunate harassment by some of the officers, and I came to realize that this just wasn't meant to be. I left law enforcement for good and went back to my other passion: working with special needs adults and kids.

This led me into a whole new career path, but one that I was already familiar with. Back home in BC I had been a swim instructor for people with disabilities and worked with a local therapeutic horseback riding program for children and adults. Due to this experience, I was able to obtain a position with the City of Ottawa in the Therapeutic Recreation Department. During the summer months, I was responsible for coordinating the integration of special needs kids into mainstream camps; during the rest of the year, I worked with Adult Recreation day programs. After some time, I started my own business helping others privately in my community, providing therapeutic recreation such as swimming lessons, outdoor activities and community integration. I also helped adults transition from living in a facility into independent living by teaching them cooking, finances, housekeeping, and medication management.

As part of this work, I was required to be certified in First Aid and CPR. I had renewed my certification so many times over the years that I decided, on top of running my own business, to become an Instructor. From there I went on to become an Instructor Trainer, teaching other people to become First Aid Instructors. I continued to teach these courses full time for about twelve years after letting go of my private business.

A turning point for my health was in 1995, when I went back home to visit my family in Vancouver. My sister and I were on our way to go shopping when a car rear-ended us so badly that my sister's car was a write-off. The man had hit the gas instead of the brakes! My seat actually broke, causing me to hit my head on the dash, and my sister crashing into the steering wheel. We were grateful to walk away from the accident though, as we knew it could have been so much worse. I discovered my injuries within the next few days. My neck and back started to ache, my range of motion was limited, and I started getting severe migraines. Little did I know this was just the beginning of a lifetime of lasting injuries and debilitating chronic pain to come. I had not yet been diagnosed with lupus, fibromyalgia, or osteoarthritis. The injuries from this accident would never really go away, becoming "non-specific connective tissue injuries"—lupus doesn't always let your body recover properly.

Another memorable moment in my life occurred a few months before François and I got married. I've always been involved in sport and exercise, even while working full time, and I wanted to keep that going into my adulthood. I was looking for an extra exercise outlet, other than just running, and discovered that there was an adult volleyball league in our neighborhood of Gatineau Quebec. It was winter and not much else going on, so I played once a week to keep in shape. One game, I jumped up to block a spike and there was a loud bang, like someone had hit the post of the net with a bat. For a whole five seconds I couldn't figure out what the sound was. Then I tried to move my left ankle; my foot looked like it was in the wrong position and my lower leg started to swell. It turns out it was the loud snapping sound we all heard was my left Achilles tendon tearing! There was no way I could walk, so even though the hospital wasn't far away we had to call an ambulance. There I was informed that I didn't just tear the tendon, I shredded it and severed it completely through. They had to surgically reattach the Achilles and repair the damage to my calf, and I was in a cast and a wheelchair for two months after. Eight months later, I managed to walk on my own on our wedding day.

I shared this story with many of my nursing students over the years as an example of communication in health care. The hospital stay was quite comical as while I spoke some French at the time, the incredible pain I was in made it nearly impossible to comprehend anything that wasn't in my native language. Once they decide I was going for surgery, they took away my glasses and I couldn't see more than some vague shapes and shadows. I could hear voices, but they were not talking to me. My senses being impaired created an enormous communication barrier, so I didn't understand much of what the doctors or nurses said. I was in excruciating pain and didn't know how to ask for pain meds in the right language. I was starving because my surgery kept getting bumped for priority patients, which is understandable but incredibly frustrating. I also wanted to use crutches to go to the bathroom; instead they brought me a commode, but I had stage fright and couldn't go unless I was behind a locked door.

Finally, after what seemed to me like an eternity of blindness, disorientation, and so much pain, I ripped out my IV, put myself onto a chair with wheels, and hurled myself down the hallway while calling out to my husband to help me. So here I was, half-on and half-off a stool, rolling down the corridor with blood dripping from my IV site, crying out for François while several nurses or orderlies chased after me. They must have thought I was insane!

François said I was in a highly drug-induced state the time, and I don't really remember all of it. But looking back on the situation makes me laugh and feel sorry for those poor nurses! What a horrible patient I had been! In my own defence, though, I was scared and in a panicked state of pain and drug-induced confusion.

My many hospitalizations and surgeries, including this one, would eventually become teaching tools and proved me with insights into the world of being a patient and a nurse, something I didn't know at the time.

After the wedding I decided I wanted more out my Emergency career, so I earned my First Responder badge and continued with my Aquatic Emergency Training. At thirty years of age I completed my Royal Life Saving, Bronze Cross, and Bronze Medallion at the University of Ottawa pool with a bunch of eighteen- to nineteen-year-old guys. They were more than a little shocked when I ended up teaching the land rescue portion of the course. These young men kicked my butt in the water, but once we were back on land it was mine turn! I started working for high-risk sporting events and taught Emergency Aquatic Rescue to the RCMP, an exciting time for me as my husband was RCMP and therefore became my student. It was fun working together!

As my Emergency Services credentials were stacking up and I was working with different age groups and different types of Emergency Agencies, I realized that this was what I was meant to do. I was helping others and living a lifetime of service. I was on my way to a fulfilling career doing what

I loved. Nothing could stop me now! Little did I know that the Universe was about to test my limits.

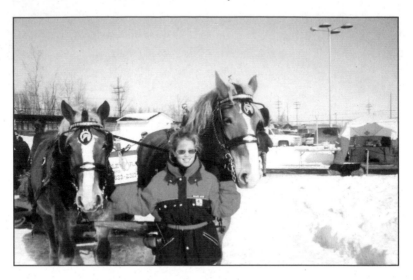

Journal reflection: Do you know what your passion is? How can you make it so this is your career and you are paid to do what you love?

_____

_____

_____

_____

Chapter 2

The diagnosis

It was January 2005, and after years of frustration I finally got a doctor to listen to me. I had been experiencing extreme fatigue and disruptive sleep, which I was told was continued postpartum depression after the birth of our son, Ben. I know what you're thinking, these are normal issues that parents face when they have a newborn, but at this point Ben was two years old! I had also been complaining about mild pain in my joints, which was dismissed as being a result of the sports I had played. While my symptoms were not affecting my day-to-day life yet, they were annoying and I wanted to figure out what was causing them.

My doctor finally sent me to a Rheumatologist who, after looking at my blood test results and my corresponding signs and symptoms, confirmed I had a mild form of systemic lupus erythematosus (SLE). I wasn't sure how to feel about this. I was terrified of the diagnosis, but on the other hand we now had a name for what was attacking my body. This meant I wasn't crazy—it wasn't all in my head.

What is lupus?

Lupus has been described as a systemic autoimmune disease or autoimmune connective tissue disease. Lupus Canada explains the condition as follows: "...in lupus, the immune system (the body's defense against viruses and bacteria) is unable to tell the difference between intruders and the body's own tissues. Trying to do its job, it attacks parts of the body, causing inflammation and creating the symptoms of lupus...Because it occurs most often in women of childbearing age, it seems evident that there is a link between lupus and some hormones, but how this works remains uncertain. It also appears that inherited factors may make certain people more likely to develop lupus, but these also are not clear yet."

Lupus is one of the most difficult diseases to diagnose due to the multitude of different symptoms that can mimic other diseases. Lupus has been nicknamed "the disease of a thousand faces", because of the complicated diagnosis process. Below are just a few of the many possible symptoms; for a diagnosis to me made, four of these should be present along with a positive blood test for Anti-Nuclear Antibodies (ANA).

1. Butterfly rash: covers the bridge of the nose and both cheeks
2. Photosensitivity: excessive skin reaction to sunlight
3. Discoid lupus: scaly red rash
4. Mucosal ulcers: small sores that line the inside of the mouth and nose
5. Arthritis: pain in the joints
6. Pleuritis or Pericarditis: inflammation of the pleura

(lining of the lungs) or the pericardium (the lining of the heart)

7. Kidney involvement: mild to serious, often fatal if not caught in early stages
8. Central Nervous System symptoms: seizures, memory loss, confusion, disorientation
9. Hemolytic anemia: disorder of the red blood cells, causes fatigue
10. Immunological disorders: way too complicated to describe here, indicated by four autoantibodies found in the blood
11. Anti-nuclear antibodies: present in the majority of people with lupus, but other symptoms must be present for a diagnosis to be confirmed

Other symptoms can be loss of hair, high blood pressure, sub-acute subcutaneous SLE, Raynaud's Phenomena, vasculitis, and severe migraines. More detailed information can be found on the Lupus Canada website.

My mosaic of symptoms

After I received my diagnosis, I did some research about systemic lupus on the internet—which I don't recommend unless you have good sources as there's a lot of scary but inaccurate information out there—and I decided I wasn't going to let this disease control my life. So, it became another challenge to overcome. My competitive nature, my drive, and my unswayable determination kicked in and away I went, carrying on like nothing had changed.

Four months after my diagnosis of SLE, my two-year-old son and I were in a car accident where we were rear-ended pretty hard. Thankfully Ben didn't have any injuries from his car seat, but I immediately experienced an aching back, stiff neck and shoulders, and severe shooting pain, weakness, and loss of range of motion in my left arm. There was no delay to the onset of my injuries this time; my body responded differently than the last accident. This is when life as I knew it would change. The impact of the crash triggered the lupus to flare up badly and attack my joints, muscles, skin, and brain.

My own symptoms have changed over the past fourteen years since my original diagnosis. They started with mostly **fatigue, general weakness and widespread pain**. **Migraines** would start coming on with a vengeance after my first TIA in 2005. Then, it started to get really scary. I would have large **blank spaces of memory loss**, where I couldn't recall recent the past months or weeks. Other times I experienced **short-term memory loss,** where I couldn't remember if I'd stopped at a stop sign while driving or how I got home. They say time flies when you're having fun; I'd like to know what they mean. I've lost so much time in the past eleven years. Conversations or events that happened two to three years ago seem like they only happened a few months ago, or not at all. The pain and fatigue have robbed me of my memory. Some I'm happy to have lost. Other memories I grieve, such as the sound of my children's voices or the feel of their little hand in mine. I would also have periods of **agitation and short-temperedness** with the frustration of not being able to have recall my memories. This is managed better now that I know what's going on.

As soon as I started on the Plaquenil (Hydrochroqueline) to suppress my overactive immune system, I became **hypertensive to the sun**, along with experiencing itchy, red rashes and severe nausea for the first six months. After a few more months the nausea got better, but I was still getting sunburns in less than five minutes even in only minimal sunlight. This kept me indoors or in the shade for the first two summers; I missed out on a lot that year. I even found I was reacting to certain indoor lights, particularly with overhead fluorescent lighting. While this has improved, I still get rashes from the sun, although they could also be from certain foods that cause inflammation or irritation, or from stress; something I need to pay more attention to.

Later, more symptoms would come forward such as a **loss of sensation in my hands and feet** as well as **numbness and tingling in my elbows, forearms, and hands**. Then my shoulder froze, and I started getting shooting pain across my upper back and into my ribcage. Eventually I would get **progressive, stabbing chest pain from the pleuritis** around my lungs, as well as **difficulty breathing** and **inflammation of the cartilage between my ribs. Foot pain** came and went with no rhyme or reason. Eventually my neck stopped turning properly, which meant I had **limited range of motion of my head**. It was difficult to hold it up right and the migraines came back.

My sacroiliac joints, which are found in the lower back, started locking up and sending **electric-like shock pain down my leg** behind my knee, and all the way to my feet, which caused my **legs to give out**.

Currently, the bursitis and osteoarthrosis in my hips are flaring up big time because I'm sitting a lot while I write this book. The **freezing of my neck and shoulder joints** is back, no doubt also from too much writing. Thank goodness my Fitbit reminds me to get up every hour and move. In the last four years I have developed **TMJ**, which is a disorder that affects the joint between your jaw and your skull. I have to manually push a spot adjacent to my ear to pop my jaw open. No more gum chewing for me, unless I have surgery. Due to the lupus I am at a **higher risk of infection and complications,** so this is not going to happen.

Sjogrens syndrome—an immune system disorder affecting the eyes and mouth—has **dried up my left salivary gland.** The orthodontic surgeon said its likely that stone build up in the gland is causing additional pain in my jaw, but once again it's too risky to operate. Something else to live with—yay for Biotene (oral hydrate rinse)! As another anomaly of the Sjogrens, sometimes **my eyes dry up or leak.** From time to time I'll wake up with some weird infection and can neither see nor get my contacts in for three days.

Over the years, **depression** would take over at times and antidepressants became part of my treatment. Battling pain and immobility every day can be an extremely lonely life to live, and there are times when all you feel is hopelessness. You end up going through a grieving process every time you lose part of your former self; it feels like you have lost a loved one you were very close to and will never see again. Take the time to recognize these difficult feelings and get some help. DO NOT TRY DO THIS ON YOUR OWN! **YOU ARE NOT ALONE!**

If you're newly diagnosed, try not to panic. This can all seem extremely overwhelming; I know, because I've been there. The best advice that I can pass on to you is not to play the "what if" game. It makes no sense to worry over potential symptoms or diagnosis that you may never get. Every patient is different and will experience a different set of symptoms.

Another illness arises

In July of the same year as my lupus diagnosis, just three days before my thirty-sixth birthday, the universe threw me another curveball. My husband and I had taken our two-and-a-half-year-old to Tofino, where we had rented a beach-front cottage along with my husband's brother and his family. One day, everyone wanted to hike out to Long Beach. I'd been feeling under the weather for at least two months beforehand, but that day I was feeling particularly strange. It was not something I could put into words at the time as I didn't realize what was happening to me. I was trying to be a good sport though, so I packed up a lunch and headed out for what was going to be a turning point in my life.

Before we left, I noticed I was feeling fatigued and low energy. But, this is not uncommon for someone with an autoimmune disease so I ignored it and trooped on. I don't have much memory of the rest of the day, and if we hadn't taken pictures I'm not sure I would remember anything at all. I do recall seeing myself sitting on a chair, wrapped in a beach blanket to protect myself from the wind. I was motionless and felt like I was outside of my body, frozen in time as I watched my husband and my young toddler play in the sand with my niece and nephew. Why was I not able to get up and run around like everyone else? I wanted to scream but nothing would come out.

The next memory I have is of us standing in a parking lot at the beach, waiting for my husband to get the car as I was not able to walk to whole way back to where we were staying. Then I see myself held up by my husband as we struggle to climb the steps of our cottage, trying to get me inside so I can lie down.

I do remember a strong tingling, almost buzzing sensation on the right side of my face as well as in my fingers and my feet. I don't really recall what my vision was doing at the time, but I do remember I couldn't form a sentence; I knew what I wanted to say, but the words were stuck and wouldn't come out. I was terrified. I was having a Transient Ischemic Attack (TIA), which is described by the Journal of the American Medical Association as "a focal disturbance of brain or retinal ischemia lasting less than twenty-four hours and without evidence of infarction." In layman's terms, it is a small, temporary or warning stroke.

As a medic and a First Aid and CPR Instructor for many years, I knew full well what was happening. That's a good thing, right? It is, if you tell someone what's happening or what to do. Instead, I did what I always do and downplayed my situation. I rested for what I thought was a few minutes, although I was told later it had been several hours. After I got up, I started to help get our crab feast underway. I knew that I really should go to the hospital in town, but that would spoil our last night together and my husband's family had travelled all the way from Quebec for this trip. Also, it was a fresh crab dinner! Who would want to miss that? I decided that I would just get through dinner and see how I felt after. Looking back, I want to kick myself!

TIAs do not cause much permanent damage to the brain; however, they often are a warning sign that a full-blown stroke may happen soon. According to the American Heart Association, "The chance of a subsequent stroke after an acute transient ischemic attack (TIA) or minor stroke is high, with a 90-day risk between 10% and 20%. The prognosis for these patients is often unfavourable." Some people have only a single occurrence, while others have recurrent episodes. It's not clear if I've had more than one since then, but I have had instances of severe sudden migraine, inability to put slurred words together to form a proper sentence, immobility and severe weakness of one side of my body and face, and more memory loss. I'm also now extremely prone to vertigo, severe migraines, and even aura migraines, which the Mayo clinic defines as "a migraine that's preceded or accompanied by a variety of sensory warning signs or symptoms, such as flashes of light, blind spots or tingling in your hand or face."

When we got back from our visit to the island, I was told I had been acting agitated and unreasonable. No one knew how sick I really was at the time, or that my mood had been altered by the lupus and the stroke. A few days later my Rheumatologist referred me to a Neurologist, and after a few weeks I went for an assessment to see if there was any permanent damage. It was determined that there was no long-lasting impairment of gross motor skills, other than some general weakness with minimal limitations with fine motor skills. However, I was demonstrating severe fatigue and short-term memory loss. They prescribed me another medication to help keep migraines to a minimum along with an antiplatelet therapy or blood thinner to prevent blood clots from reoccurring.

Having any kind of stroke is always considered an emergency! It's important for you and your family members to be aware of the signs and symptoms of stroke and heart attack, as well as having CPR training, so you have a plan of action when an emergency presents itself. This will hopefully give the person affected a better chance of survival, and gives some peace of mind for you and your loved ones.

Journal reflection: How prepared is your family for a medical emergency?

_____

_____

_____

_____

Chapter 3

Finding your health care team

Before I go any further, I want to take the opportunity to say wholeheartedly that I now have an amazing team of doctors and specialists that I see on a regular basis. My GP, Rheumatologist, Chiropractor, and Massage Therapist—along with several other specialists that I see—are caring, compassionate, respectful, open-minded, and professional. I wouldn't be here today without their close attention to detail regarding my complicated illnesses and their encouragement to keep getting better. Thank you Dr. I., Dr. A., Dr. W., and Ms. M.! I love you all!

As a nurse, I can tell you that most doctors are extremely compassionate and have your best interest at heart. However, some are so jaded that they have forgotten the lost art of bedside manner. Most patients I have met who live with chronic illness have had more than a few unpleasant experiences with a medical professional such as a family doctor or specialist. They are usually a bit hesitant to seek help from their family doctor, especially if their symptoms are associated with an invisible illness, because they feel like they are being judged.

This situation is especially tricky for nurses or other medical professionals as we already have a self-diagnosis in mind. We know what information that the doctor is looking for, so we are somewhat prepared for the onslaught of questions that are used as a process of elimination to reach a diagnosis. The trouble is that we professionals sometimes have too much information, which can lead to a confrontation, depending on the personality of your family doctor—also referred to as a general practitioner or GP—as well as your own approach to the subject at hand. Nurses are notorious for not taking very good care of ourselves—especially female nurses who are also moms—and for not being the best patients.

Sometimes doctors don't respond well to having a nurse as a patient. When I go to see a new doctor or specialist, my background in nursing has often been received with one of two responses. Either the doctor is impressed and thrilled that they don't have to spend a lot of time explaining an illness or disease process. Or, they are offended and become defensive or threatened by another medical professional and feel that, by expressing my knowledge on the subject, I am questioning their authority. The latter response is disappointing and frustrating to encounter. I'm no doctor, but I certainly don't expect to be talked down to. After these experiences, I now avoid mentioning that I was a nurse and just keep this information to myself.

Why I fired my former doctor

Typically, I tend to wait until something is a significant problem before I seek medical attention from anyone. In other words, I often will ignore symptoms for weeks or months before I make an appointment with my doctor. It's not always the smart approach, but its forever intimidating to make that call once one doctor says there's nothing wrong with you or that it's all in your head. Sometimes, doctors don't take you seriously or don't believe what you are saying. You already don't feel well or are stressed about a possible diagnosis, and for the doctor to assume you are making things up is so disrespectful and disheartening. It makes you feel like a fool, when really you just want to be well and move on with your life. My anxiety goes up just thinking about it. Often my excuse is that I already know what they are going to say, and usually I'm right or at least pretty darn close.

I am aware that some people exaggerate their symptoms and play the victim for attention; I've even experienced it with my own patients. Typically, these patients are either lonely or suffering from some sort of mental health issue, and their situation deserves to be addressed either way. People need to be treated with respect, regardless of their reason for seeking help.

For instance, on one occasion my former GP and I discovered a lump in my left breast. She referred me to go for a mammogram, and once the results were in I was called in for an appointment to discuss the findings. When I got there, my doctor seemed to be agitated by the fact that I had told the radiology technician there was a lump. She questioned me why I would say that, and my response was simple: because we both had found a lump, which is why she had referred me to get the mammogram in the first place. Her frustration made no sense to me; she was making me feel like I had made the whole thing up. At this point the doctor finally looked at my file, after which she sheepishly agreed with me and stated she had forgotten. If she had simply trusted what I said, or even taken time to look at my file in advance, we would have had a pleasant appointment rather than one where I was left feeling like she didn't believe me.

Another time, I had a specialist accuse me of being a cocaine addict because of the lesions in my nose. I told him I was a nurse, and he responded that this was all the more reason for his concern about my so-called addiction. I explained that I had been kicked in the face playing rugby in high school and had to have reconstructive surgery on my nasal septum, and this never healed properly and became an added site of constant irritation because of my lupus. A rheumatologist should be acutely aware that most patients with SLE don't recovery well or as fast from injuries, but he just smirked at me and continued to write notes. I left his office in tears, but I was proud that I had refrained from calling him out for being the jerk that he was. It wouldn't have been productive, but it sure would have felt good!

A third doctor told me I was a "basket case." She had pegged me as a very nervous person and was basically indicating that I was a hypochondriac. I was floored, insulted, and furious. I said to her, "but you only see me when I'm not feeling well. Why not meet for a beer at the pub and you get to see me when I'm well." I was angry, and of course then I started second guessing myself, which I shouldn't be doing. I barely see my GP unless something is really wrong. Could you imagine if I went in for everything that was wrong with me, with all the symptoms from all my chronic illnesses? I'd be there every day and then I'd have to start paying rent!

I fired all three of these doctors and found ones who treated me with respect. Don't waste your time on medical professionals who are not committed to helping you get better.

It's okay to look for someone that will hear you and show you the compassion and respect you deserve!

My advice on patient advocacy

Your relationship with your medical team should be a partnership; there should be an exchange of communication that both parties understand. I must tell you there are some amazing healthcare professionals out there who genuinely care and are concerned for your wellbeing. However, they can't help if you are not honest about how you are feeling. *You* are responsible for your own health care!

The squeaky wheel gets the grease. Be honest about your symptoms, but flaunt the ones you have and milk them for all they're worth! Make sure you're heard and don't downplay what you are experiencing. If you have to go to an emergency department, they're going to ask you a lot of questions; give them the brutal truth! If you have pain, be specific. Is it sharp, stabbing, aching, throbbing, floating, deep, narrow, constant, comes and goes, only hurts if you move a certain way, only if pressure is applied, and how bad it is on a scale of 1-10? Does it hurt more if you stay still or if you move? Can you use heat or ice? Do you need to elevate an arm or leg? Are you experiencing difficulty breathing, do you have chest pain, are you on any medication, and when was your last meal and what did you eat? When your last bowel movement, and what size and shape was it? Make sure you know your symptoms are (what you feel), in the event that your signs (what they see) are not as present. With all that being said, NEVER fake a symptom; this ruins your credibility as a patient and makes it harder for you—and for others in your situation—to get the treatment you need. It's also incredibly disruptive of our already understaffed and overworked health care teams.

Take notes about your symptoms. People with multiple chronic illnesses face additional difficulties when visiting the doctor. It can be a struggle to try and remember how or when symptoms started, as they tend to overlap or come as a secondary symptom from something else. Then at your appointment, you feel stupid as you are humming and hawing, trying to remember what it was you were going to say. I always recommend writing your symptoms down, but then I forget to do it myself. Typical nurse; the rules don't apply to us, only to the other patients!

When researching your symptoms, make sure that you are getting your information from a reliable source, such as well-known medical sites or university studies. Never simply consult Doctor Google about your symptoms; he can give you very inaccurate information, which almost always leads to a prognosis of death. Not all information we get from the internet is accurate, and misinformed search results can send you off on a misleading wild goose chase where you may get the wrong answers. Make sure you're looking at a credible site; I recommend using government-registered disease awareness charities and university medical links.

Don't believe everything your friends tell you. Don't assume that because your friend Joe's cousin's uncle's wife had the same illness that your diagnosis or prognosis will be the same. There is always someone with a story of some relative with similar symptoms to what you are experiencing; however, you may have the same symptoms but coming from a different type of illness. There are literally thousands of illnesses that mimic each other. On the other hand, you can have the same condition as someone else, but have completely different symptoms. There is also the possibility that two people have the exact same illness but may be treated differently. This is all part of factoring in any pre-existing medical conditions (such as high blood pressure, diabetes, or lupus), age, mobility, cognitive behavior, medication, gender, and family history. Who's to know for sure if your friend or family member has all the right information in the first place, or where they got it from?

Be knowledgeable about the treatments for your condition. Look for options that are safe, easily accessible, and have a good success rate. Check to see if your medications have a generic form, which is often significantly cheaper, and what brands are covered by your insurance. Also, it is important that you are aware of the probability of outcome, meaning the risks involved as a result of your treatment.

Get a second opinion. If you're not sure that your doctor is knowledgeable on your condition, or if they are not investigating your symptoms, you need to go elsewhere where you will be heard. As I mentioned above, I have personally fired three doctors. I needed to feel confident that I was in good care, that I was being heard, and that my best interests were first and foremost. I did finally find an excellent GP, whom by the way is also a teaching physician. Dr. Evaristus Idanwekhai, MBBS,CFFB listens to me and is up to date on recent studies that relate to all of my many odd illnesses.

You should also keep in mind, though, that there are limits to what your GP can do. GP stands for General Practitioner. That means they are practicing general medicine, not specializing in anything. When there is something your doctor is unclear on and they have exhausted all of their own diagnostics and resources, they should be sending you to a specialist. That's how our system is supposed to work. My Rheumatologist, Dr. Antonio Avina-Zubetia, is probably the most educated, kind, and genuine and medical professional I've ever met. He listens, he's compassionate, but he also doesn't let things go by the way side. He's very proactive in my care and makes sure I've had the proper diagnostic tests, follows up on my blood work, and makes sure my pain is under control.

It's wonderful and heart-warming to know that your doctors are supportive of your healing in all aspects of your life and not just your pain. Both my new GP and Rheumy have been instrumental at getting my pain under control and making sure my mental health is receiving attention just as much as my physical wellbeing. I trust them both with my life.

But, it took a long time—and a lot of frustrating and upsetting medical appointments—for me to find the right health care team.

Those of us with chronic illnesses want to get better and have a "normal life" like other people do. We want to get dressed and go to work and go hiking and be able to sit or stand to enjoy a concert or hockey game. We'd like to do all these things without having to strategize about every aspect of the day. What clothes can I get on by myself? What shoes will allow for the swelling I will experience three hours from now? What pain meds can I take, or can I take any at all? How am I getting there and back? Can I drive myself, or if I need pain meds who can I ask to take me? Is there a bathroom nearby? Will there be sunshine or heat or cold? Will there be bright lights or loud noises that could trigger a migraine? The list is endless. If I'm experiencing a flare up, I have to deal with symptoms like severe fatigue, muscle weakness, neuropathy (nerve pain), migraines, nausea, dizziness, digestive disorders, joint pain, inflammation, neck and back pain, widespread aching and stabbing pain, brain fog, memory loss, loss of balance, insomnia, anxiety, difficulty breathing, chest pain, immobility, and limited range of motion. All of which get in the way of living the life that I desperately want to live.

This is why I get angry when some doctor questions the validity of my symptoms. How dare they assume I hadn't thought this through? The constant fear of judgement is one of the main reasons chronically ill patients end becoming reclusive and refusing to leave the house. Trying to appear "normal" is more work than being authentically sick; it's so much easier to stay home where no one is around to judge.

Might I point out at this time that for those chronically ill people that do manage to "get out," let me tell you, we are fierce warriors! We are masters at making debilitating pain and illness vanish from sight so as not to draw attention to it. We hide behind words like "I'm fine," "I'm okay," or "I'm good" so we can avoid the unsolicited advice we are sick of hearing. But we also do it to protect others, for fear of upsetting them, because we don't ever want anyone to suffer as much as we have. It would be unbearable. So instead, we carry this burden in silence.

At a time when I'm feeling judgement, which is usually on a daily basis, I turn to one of my favorite scriptures:

"Who I am in Christ matters more than what I think or what others tell me about myself."
Colossians 3:1-4 (NIV)

Journal reflection: Are you and your health care practitioner a team? Do you have the same goals in mind for your health?

_____

_____

_____

_____

Chapter 4

Tips for the hospital stay

A week before Christmas I was experiencing pain in the left side of my lower back, which I recognized as being a kidney stone. I usually pass them at home, but this time I passed a rather large blood clot which we assume contained the stone, or at least part of it. Shortly after, I started experiencing shock-like symptoms. My temperature spiked, my blood pressure dropped, and my heart rate was way above what it should be. My lips were bluish and I was shaking uncontrollably and slightly confused. The strangest symptom was the all-over body pain; my skin hurt to touch. My husband and my dad knew something was wrong with me, so they decided to take me to the hospital.

When we got to the ER, it took them four or five tries to finally get an IV started as my veins were uncooperative. They put me on oxygen and started monitoring my heart rate. My oxygen saturation levels were dipping into the eighties on room air; the average person should be at least ninety-five. I wasn't critical but, needless to say, I was not well at all. They were suspecting sepsis, which means your kidneys are no longer filtering out toxins properly, causing them to leak out into your blood stream. This condition can be a deadly if not treated quickly.

I was at the hospital for two days while we waited two days for the antibiotics to kick in. At this point I was no longer a cardiac risk and was breathing adequately on my own, so they took me off the oxygen and told me I would be moved to a medical unit for further testing and IV antibiotic treatments. They had no room for me that day, so I was going to be put out in a hallway; unfortunately, this is not an uncommon practice in the overloaded BC healthcare system. The next available room was a four-bed room. Two of the patients in this room had behavioral tendencies, which is a polite way of saying they moan and scream all day. My bigger concern, though, was the third patient, who was on "contact precaution." This means that the patient either came in with an infectious disease that is spreadable by direct or indirect contact, or they have acquired it during their hospital stay.

Know your rights as a patient

Situations such as this one illustrate why it's important to know your rights as a patient. The hospital is not a prison, nor is it a hotel. You do have some options, although they are limited at best. As soon as I heard about the infection risk, I put the brakes on. No way am I going into a room where there is a strong potential for me to get even sicker than I already am. I'm fighting a serious kidney infection and I already have a compromised immune system due to my systemic lupus. Let's not make it harder for me to recover by adding in another serious infection.

The charge nurse explained to me that the patients rarely get out of bed and I really shouldn't worry about them. I explained to her as politely as I could that I wasn't so much worried about the patient with the contact precaution as I was with the nursing staff and the family visitors. I can say this because I've worked in the hospital, and I've witnessed firsthand a small handful of nurses who neither change their gloves nor wash their hands between patients. Don't get me wrong, most nurses are excellent at maintaining proper hygiene to prevent the spread of infections. However, sometimes when it gets busy, a few nurses may bypass this precaution or occasionally forget. Worse yet, family members that are visiting a patient in isolation are not being taught the proper protocols for contact or airborne diseases. They are sitting on the bed or using the bathrooms intended for the patient, and therefore inadvertently make contact with whatever superbug the patient is fighting. That family member is now spreading it around the unit, bringing into their car and their home, and sharing it with their family members.

Here's the tip: you have the right to refuse treatment and to refuse the room they put you in. You do not, however, get to choose when or where you will go, which puts you—or in this case, me—back in the hallway. The charge nurse argued that by staying in the hallway I was already in an uncontrolled environment. I disagreed. The next room that came available was a two-bed room, and the other patient was not under contact precaution warning. I spent the next day in this room as I waited to finally be released to go home; if, of course, the doctors could agree on what to do with me. There were two hospitalists, an internal medicine doctor, a urology med student, and three infectious disease specialists all weighing in on what should happen to me, and they did not all agree on the severity of my symptoms.

Another important tip: do you feel well enough to go home with the medications provided? Are you capable of taking care of yourself? Can you stand, walk, and go to the bathroom on your own? Are you no longer considered a critical patient? If so, then you are ready to go home! The hospital is the worst place for a stable patient to recover. You'll get more rest and sleep without all the necessary disruptions and noise made by the nursing staff and other patients and their families, as well as less exposure to communicable diseases.

The medical team as a whole never reached a consensus on whether or not I should be discharged. With all the different diseases fighting in my body, my situation was extremely complicated. Eventually the infectious disease doctors, the evening hospitalist doctor, and I decided that because I was no longer in need of oxygen or nursing care, I could take oral antibiotics at home. There were still a lot of blood work pending, as well as a follow up appointment with my Urologist and a cystoscopy to determine if the infections were starting in the bladder or in the kidney.

It is important that you are an active participant in your own health care. You are ultimately responsible for knowing your body and keeping your medical information up to date. That means knowing what your medications are, being able to describe your symptoms accurately, and understanding that each person you come across does not always have your medical information on hand; you may have to repeat your information a few times to different people. On the flip side of this, you have a right to know what diagnostic tests they are performing, what the results are, what the treatment and prognosis is, and if there are other options available to you. Don't be afraid to ask questions; it's your body, and it's your right to know!

The cranky nurse

If you are in a hospital, you will likely end up coming across a cranky nurse or doctor. One thing that you need to remember in this situation is that they are only human. It's also important to note that nurses have one the most stressful workplace environments.

As a former surgical nurse, I can tell you that a twelve-hour shift can make some of the most kind and caring people bend under the pressures that have been put on them. Looking back on my career, I can honestly say that I was not always able to give each patient 100% of my best effort due to the unrealistic expectations placed on me by our overcrowded hospitals.

I always started a shift with the intention of giving my patients all of the care and attention they deserved, but the system would constantly get in the way. Our much-needed breaks were often cut short because a patient was in crisis or we were short-staffed. The units are often overloaded, and we couldn't keep up with the intake assessments, treatments, bloodwork, medications, toileting, feeding, dressing, surgical wound care, IV maintenance, post-op recovery, vitals, repositioning, intake and output of fluids, and discharging of patients, just to mention a few of our responsibilities. We also needed to document every single thing we did and report on for four to six patients per nurse. If your partner was on break, you were accountable for his or her patients as well as your own.

I miss my coworkers and I miss my patients, but I certainly don't miss the chaos. Our medical system is overcrowded, mostly because our population continues to grow. The pressure of caring for an ever-increasing number of patients falls on the entire health care team, but as primary caregivers nurses take a large portion of this burden. A huge part of the problem is that there is an insane amount of people going to the hospital who instead should be going to their family doctor or walk-in clinic.

While were on this subject, lets address what warrants a visit to the Emergency department. Cold and flu-like symptoms can be treated at home or at a clinic. There's not much you can do for a cold other than wait it out and maybe take something to help alleviate symptoms; any pharmacist can help you with this. Choose the no-name brand over-the-counter medicine as it usually has the exact same medicinal ingredients without the brand-name price tag.

Some of the signs and symptoms that warrant going to emergency are bleeding that won't stop, persistent chest pain, difficulty breathing, diabetic emergency, blocked kidney stones, inexplicable and intense pain, or if your doctor has directed you to go to Emergency for any reason. If you're unsure where you should go, you can always contact your local public health nurse and ask.

By avoiding going to the emergency room for non-urgent health concerns, you help reduce the load placed on the hospital staff and allow the patients who do need emergency care to get what they need.

Let's be clear: there are a few nurses or doctors that may have chosen the wrong profession, or who have simply have burned out and need to move on. Most nurses, however—including myself—*love* what they do! They are some of the most intelligent, adaptive, resourceful, caring, loving, nurturing, attentive, responsible, strong, and kind-hearted people you'll ever know. They are also some of the bravest warriors in health care due to the high risk of violence and abuse in their workplace. On top of all this, they are constantly being overworked, which is an epidemic we need to be aware of.

So, the next time you must visit the hospital or clinic, please keep in mind us nurses are only human, and we are doing the best we can with what have to work with. The system is broken, and that has a huge impact on the incredible people that work within it. The best way to show your appreciation and support for your health care team is to remember to thank them! Say thank you to the unit clerk that got your file started; the porter that wheeled you to your treatment area and helped you into a hospital gown; the nurse that did your vitals and assessment, gave you your pain meds, and performed other treatments; the lab tech that did your blood work; the doctor that gave you your diagnosis and determined the next steps in your care; and, last but not least, the maintenance crew that picked up the garbage. Yes, even the maintenance crew! They're an amazing team, and our hospitals would not run without them.

Journal reflection: How much of your life do you "fake" being well to please others?

_____

_____

_____

_____

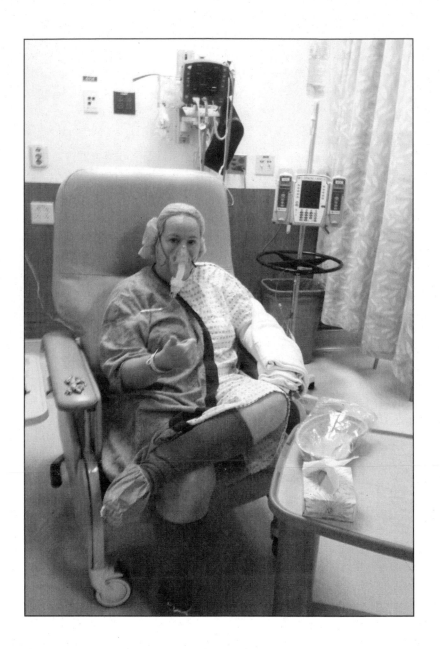

Chapter 5

Adventures and PTSD

Most of my life has been an adventure. I had that need for speed—that determination to do high-adrenaline, difficult work—that took me on exhilarating and challenging journeys. I wanted to save the world.

In 1998, I trained in Critical Incident Stress Management and traveled south to work as a member of the Disaster Response Hurricane George Relief Team. I was given twenty-four hours to book a flight, grab my passport, pack a small suitcase, scribble out a hand-written will just in case, and notify my family and work that I would be gone for up to six weeks. I wasn't sure where my posting was, other than that it was somewhere in Puerto Rico. Just before heading to the airport, I went for my briefing along with two local firefighters who were also being deployed to the same area. During our long flight, we quickly became fast friends and shared stories of our loved ones, day jobs, hobbies, and how each of us had gotten onto the International Disaster Response Team (DRT) for the Canadian Red Cross.

Upon arrival at the San Juan airport, we were escorted to the Disaster Headquarters. There we were met by local members of the disaster team, American Red Cross, and AmeriCorps. People were running in and out of the building, shouting orders and grabbing maps and water. It was total chaos. I was separated from my firefighter friends and sent to Mayaguez. I spent the next several hours driving with total strangers who didn't speak much English, and I spoke almost no Spanish whatsoever.

San Juan was cleaned up fairly quickly as the city relies heavily on their tourism industry. The countryside, however, was still in pretty bad shape. Most of the fields were flooded, fences were wiped out, dead and decaying animals lay on the side of the road, and livestock roamed free. One of the saddest sights, which I will never forget, was that of a dog sitting on the side of the road alongside another dog, who was already deceased. He or she sat beside this poor creature for days on end, mourning its passing, hoping it would awake and rise. This image still haunts me when I think of those days.

The hurricane winds had uprooted most of the palm trees and washed out major roads, limiting access to the people up in the mountains. When I reached my local disaster headquarters in Mayaguez, I found out that those mountain people would become my responsibility. After checking in with my supervisor I was introduced to the other members of the team, which included nurses, paramedics, firefighters, and military. My assignment was to go into the mountains to assess what was needed, which turned out to be food, water, clothing, cooking utensils, pots, pans, and medical attention.

I have no idea how these people were able to survive for

the past two weeks before our crew showed up to help. The ones who did have a vehicle could go to the makeshift disaster depot at the local airport and get food, water, clothing, and medical attention. But those without the transportation or gas to get there were stranded up in the mountains without help. I quickly got into a routine with my team and my translator, getting these people the assistance they needed.

I shared a room with a nurse from the US. We didn't always see each other out in the field, but at the end of the day—which could sometimes be twelve to fourteen hours long—we made sure to check how we were doing. We called it a "mini mental" or a "quick head check," and it helped us ensure we were still able to do our jobs without becoming secondary victims of what we saw and heard.

One evening, we were woken up by the sound of shouting in the courtyard outside our window. A security guard, who earlier that day had followed us to our room to make sure we arrived back safely, was now in a drunken rage and wanted everyone to know it. Earlier, he had quite publicly announced to our team that he found me to be the most beautiful white girl he had ever seen, and that he wanted to marry me. We had all laughed at the time because we thought he was joking. Apparently, he wasn't. I heard the sound of rocks hitting our window, and then the phone rang. I picked it up as my roommate came out of her room to see what was going on, and on the other end of the line was a team member who was whisper-shouting, "get down on the floor, he's got a gun!" Turns out the rocks we heard were actually gun shots aimed in our direction. We both stumbled as I dragged my roommate to the floor, silencing her with my finger to my mouth. We were panicking and wanted to call security, but we couldn't. He was security! Luckily for us, the man eventually passed out. We barely slept all night, and by morning we were exhausted. We informed the manager of the motel about our evening shoot-out serenade, and thankfully we had a new security guard the next night who didn't drink on the job or make any marriage proposals.

The days were filled with misunderstood translating, terrible fast food, frustration at the of lack of supplies, and the feeling that we weren't doing enough for these mountain people. I was only supposed to be doing family and household assessments to determine how many people had survived and whether they had the necessary supplies. However, so many of the survivors had been struck by flying debris or crushed by furniture and left with open sores, deep lacerations, contusions, fractures, and infections. How could I go all the way up there, knowing they needed wound care, and not take care of them? I just couldn't turn and walk away.

I would finish my habitat assessment, then clean and treat as many of the injured as I could before I had to head back. Word got out that there was a "healer" from Canada, and before long I had a following. Crowds would swarm the truck I was in and children would follow me, grab my hand, and ask to come with them to help their injured or sick loved ones. Often my translator and I would lose track of time and be late heading back into town. I was called out a few times on our radio frequency for not heading back before dark, especially if rain came because the roads would wash out easily. We would hear, "that Canadian girl, still taking her time up that mountain. What is taking her so long anyway?"

It wasn't long before my supervisor got word of what we were doing and realized that this is why I was always late getting back to base at night. He wasn't happy, but he turned a blind eye and pretended he didn't know what was going on. We secretly stocked up on first aid supplies to help the wounded and candies for the to give to the children that I couldn't help; there just wasn't enough time or supplies to see everyone. For the people I couldn't reach, we would encourage neighbors to check on them.

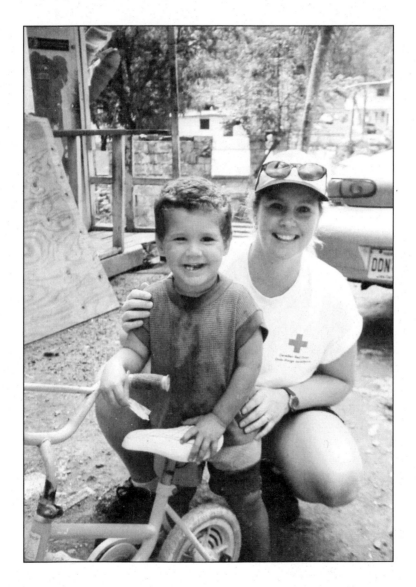

I spent the entire month of November in Puerto Rico, desperately missing my family but fiercely proud of the coordinated efforts our DRT team had made. It would not be until my return later in December that I would have my first known experience with Post-Traumatic Stress Disorder (PTSD). I was at the grocery store with my husband, and as soon as we hit the produce aisle I lost it. All the fresh fruit and vegetables, right beside the freshly baked bread, looked and smelled so amazing! I was suddenly hit with a wave of grief for the people I had left behind in Mayaguez with barely any food all. How could we have so much abundance here and not realize how lucky we are to live like this?

In 1999, I served with the Canadian Red Cross DRT at two military bases in Canada, where we received five thousand refugees from Kosovo. This amazing humanitarian operation would also become my second experience with PTSD.

My first posting was as a Volunteer Coordinator at the military base in Trenton, Ontario. My duty was to recruit, train, and organize all of the volunteers for the entire operation. I would also act as liaison between the military pastor and our DRT team; I didn't know this at the time, but he would play a big part in my search for faith and God. We met almost every day during our coffee break to communicate updates on the refugees and the volunteers. He would pray over me and my team—something new for me, but it left me with a profound feeling of protection and love. We'd discuss how amazing it was that so many people had gifted their time to make this operation the success it was, and how it truly was a blessing to be part of this international humanitarian cause.

After a few weeks our team was solid and running smoothly, so I was transferred over to the base in Borden as the Reunification Coordinator. My job here was one of the most rewarding experiences of my life. I interviewed refugees to find out who was with them here at the base, if they were missing family members, and if they knew where their family might be. Many of the refugees literally didn't know where they were. Where was Canada, was it close to their home in Kosovo? I had to register them with the Red Cross Identification program, which was created by the International Committee of the Red Cross (ICRC), whose mission is to "protect the life and dignity of the victims of international and internal armed conflicts."

One problem I encountered was that these refugees came from a culture where not many women held positions of power and influence. No one wanted to speak to me because they thought it would be a waste of their time. How could a woman possible help them to locate family at the other end of the world? I sat in my office at the base, staring at the empty doorway, completely frustrated. We were supposed to be helping these people, but how can I do that if they won't come to see me!

Eventually, my staff and I came up with idea. My translator somehow spread a rumour that made my last name, "Cadotte," sounded or looked like the Albanian word for "soldier." The next day I had a line up that was half an hour long. I didn't care what they thought my last name meant—I could finally do my job!

Once the registration was completed, we would input the family information into the ICRC system and send it to Geneva. Then, we would wait see if other family members had been registered somewhere else in the world. It is quite an amazing operation. My very first match came quickly; I received a message from the ICRC that they had located some family members at refugee camp in Germany. We took the message to our immigration staff, where it was cleared of any war content, and then I was free to approach the family and give them the good news. They had family that were alive and well!

My next match will always hold a special place in my heart. As I mentioned earlier, I had already worked at the refugee camp at the Trenton base and gotten to know some of the families that we had received. One particular man stood out for some reason, and I asked him to write a message in hope we could locate his brother and his family. He didn't know if he was dead or alive, or where in the world he might have ended up; refugees had been displaced and sent to other parts of Europe, the US, and Canada. Many of the refugees had similar last names, but for some reason I had a strong hunch that this man's family was nearby. I had his message screened by immigration, got in my car, and drove three hours back to the base in Trenton. It turned out my hunch was right! I found this man's brother and his family safe and sound, only a few hundred miles away. I then had the brother write a return message, had it screened, and keep my fingers crossed. The next day I drove back to camp at Base Borden and I arranged for the family to meet. I'll never forget the look on the man's face when I gave him the news. There were tears of joy and screams of excitement from his pregnant wife and two children. He collapsed to his knees and thanked me. I had the honour of being at the hospital to visit them when his wife gave birth to their third child, which was the first refugee born on the base camp. The baby grew up in a safe and happy environment, and her parents and older sister kept in touch with me for years to come, sending pictures and letters and reminiscing of our time shared at the refugee camp. I will always hold a special place in my heart for them.

But, the story doesn't end here. I carried scars from

my adventure home with me and into my dreams. While working in family reunification, I had to send one of my team member's home as she was displaying classic signs of traumatic stress: hyper-alertness (exaggerated startle response), trouble concentrating, and avoiding tasks that triggered anxiety. This came from being exposed to the refugees' stories of their recent escape from their war-torn country. Secondary traumatic stress is quite common among disaster team members, although not many will talk about it. There were sickening accounts of humiliation, kidnapping, rape, bombing, execution, hiding, and eventual escape.

My own nightmares started to haunt me while I was at the military base in Borden, Ontario. I don't sleep well away from home to begin with, but the exhaustion I felt after long days of interviewing refugees meant that sleep came easily. At first, I thought the dreams were just a reflection of what happened during my day. A woman I had registered would come to me in the darkness of my room with her youngest child on her hip, the older child standing beside her, holding her mother's hand and half hiding behind her skirt. The three of them would stand at the end of my bed in the dead of night, looking pale and malnourished, urging me to wake. The mother was begging me in Albanian to find her husband. He had been kidnapped by the soldiers. She took her children into the mountains to hide for days. When they felt it was safe, they returned to their village only find their home had been burned to the ground. They were taken to a refugee camp and then to me at the military base. I was their last hope of finding him.

I would wake in a frightened state and feel a sense of remorse for not being able to find her husband. The next day I would make contact with Geneva again for any hope that they may provide in finding him somewhere in the world, wondering if his wife and children were alive and safe.

We weren't allowed to stay deployed more than six to eight weeks at a time, with the hope that this would protect us from experiencing second-hand trauma. For me, it was too late; I was already showing the signs and symptoms of PTSD, although I wouldn't come to recognize this until years later. The Red Cross did provide us with a standard debrief when we left, but it doesn't make the memories go away.

I continue to experience PTSD, not just from these events but also from my own illnesses and relapses. Every time I have to tell someone my medical history or fill out a patient history form and write down all my prescription medications and the dosages—all six of them, plus my numerous vitamins and supplements which I think are now out numbering the prescriptions—as well as all of the hospital visits, treatments, and infections, I go through all the negative emotions that are attached to the illness or the surgery or the realization that I have gone through a lot of shit and it's not over. Mentally going through and writing out this information takes forever, not to mention the difficulty of trying to remember everything in the first place. Every time I have to do this, I feel like I'm reliving these horrible days over again. Even writing this book, I've had to step away for a few days to recover from the multiple images left in my brain.

Our brains remember pain, which can cause all kinds of problems with disease and chronic pain. This is one of the main culprits for neurological pain like you see in fibromyalgia. Its' important to talk about what you're going through and make sure you have a support network in place for the tough days. I have great friends that pray for us, bring us meals, and listen whenever we need a shoulder. It's been fourteen years of this crap, but I wouldn't have discovered who our real friends are

without having gone through it all. We definitely count our
blessings!

> **Journal reflection:** Do you have a support network in place
> to help you deal with traumatic incidents?
>
> _____
>
> _____
>
> _____
>
> _____

Chapter 6

How illness affects your family

As part of my preparation for this book, I sent out a questionnaire to a few other lupus patients and their families in hopes to discover the impact on families living with chronic illness. While I have compiled the answers below, I want to show you the response from my husband, François, to give you a different perspective on my story.

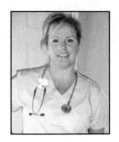

1. **What diagnosis(es) does your family member have?**
   Systemic lupus, fibromyalgia, and arthritis.

2. **Can you describe some of the symptoms they are suffering with?**
   At times unexplainable muscle and joint pain, fatigue, headaches and migraines, memory issues, and debilitating illnesses.

3. **Are you aware of the limitations this person has on any given day?**
   Yes, every day is different. One day she is fine, the other(s) not so much to very bad. The bad days overtake the good ones.

4. **Are you aware of the losses this person has experienced and why?**
   Yes, she gave up her nursing career and her ability to participate in the sports she loved due to fatigue, pain, and illnesses of all sorts. She also gave up on some of her family duties such as attending sports and school events for both her sons. Also, her share of chores within the household has significantly diminished along with personal social events.

5. **Have you done any of your own research to better understand your family member, or do you simply rely on your family member for information?**
   Yes, I have researched online in both English and French and also read a few articles and books on the subject in English. I also rely on Leisa's account on how she is doing on any given day. I do accompany her to

most medical appointments and ask the medical staff questions and also try to answer their questions when need be.

6. **Do you think this family member suffers from mental health issues because of their chronic illness? And do you know if they are receiving any assistance with this?**

If depression is a mental health issue then yes, she suffers from it, and yes, she receives help for it in the form of medication. She has also received counselling for it in the past. She also tries to make herself better by staying as active as possible (mentally and physically) and interacting with as many people as possible. She also surrounds herself with positive vibes/feel good things and people.

7. **Can you describe what types of family events that this person missed out on due to illness?**

Many of her husband and son's sports and social activities (school concerts, university graduation, hockey games and practices, Christmas office parties, family beach day, dog walks, regular family sit-down meals, etc.).

8. **How do you feel this person is managing their illness/ pain/ mental health? Could they be doing something differently?**

I believe the above-noted issues could be managed a tiny bit better at times. Let me explain: the task that lies on Leisa to get better should not be left entirely for her to manage. Immediate members of the family—such as me, her sons, father, mother, and siblings—and dear friends should take greater part in her recovery/stability. We should be able to do the simplest things such as reminding her to take her medications or pushing her a little harder to exercise when she is physically capable to do so but not ready mentally. We should put her first in our thoughts as we start our day and check on her throughout the day. Leisa is doing her best, taking into account what she has to go through on a regular basis. If one or two or three days she is not managing her illness the appropriate way, I would just commonly call it a "time off," just like regular folks need one or two or three days to relax and recover, or maybe we (the family and friends) have been forgetting about her! I believe Leisa has done and used everything in her power, short of flying to the jungle to see a voodoo doctor, to assist her in dealing with her illness. Praying to the Lord has also been a great help.

9. **How do you feel about the treatment they are receiving, and do you feel they are better and should be working on a regular/ part time basis?**

I feel that due to the strange nature of the disease, the treatments and medications available in this day and age are as good as they come. Some of the medication taken by Leisa cause weight gain, thus contributing in part to her depression. The new medical marijuana that Leisa is trying now seems to have better positive effects then others in her repertoire. But, then again, a side effect of it is that gives her the munchies

10. **Would you like to see your family member receive a different sort of treatment/help, if so why?**

Of course, but is there one? We are in pain when she is in pain, and we are down when she is! We want her to get better, plain and simple.

11. **How do you see this has affected your family member's children?**

As for my sons, they have experienced disappointment due to their mom not being able to attend important events in their lives. On a positive note, they have acquired the ability to understand and appreciate the suffering that close family members and people in general are experiencing, and how life cannot be what we expect from it all the times.

12. **Has your family member's illness affected you personally, and if so, how?**

I personally miss having her around sometimes when I would like to do something as a couple. Even when we get to do something together, most of the time it is cut short due to her suddenly falling ill. The biggest lesson I have learned from all this is that selfishness is not my friend anymore! I probably will have to take care of Leisa for the rest of my life, and that's okay with me. It's a feel-good feeling that I never understood before. She lets me know when I make a difference in her day, not only through words but by looks and touch. I have learned to be more patient and loving, which I was lacking quite a bit before the diagnoses. I am not perfect all the time and never will be, but this has changed me for the better!

Je t'aime,
François

~

Reading this made my heart melt! He gets it. It took him a while, to tell the truth, but he came around a lot faster than most. I'm so blessed! My kids, my parents, my sister, and other family members have been rock stars too. They are always encouraging and full of love and support, but there was one occasion that hit hard.

I recall one of my many nighttime visits to the hospital for some kind of flare up. I was hooked up to oxygen and IV fluids and full of pain meds. This was a few years back, as Ben wasn't old enough to stay at home by himself yet. It was a night I'll never forget. It was passed his bedtime, but we had no other choice but to bring him along as it was too late to call a babysitter. He sat on the edge of my hospital bed in his pajamas and, looking up at me with his tired little face, asked me if I was going to die. I choked back tears and tried to keep my face straight and not let him see my own fear. I don't remember exactly what I told him, other than not to worry and that I would be going home soon. It broke my heart to think about how scared my little boy must have been, seeing his mommy sick like that. I wished he didn't have to keep going through this. On the positive side, I know other lupus patients with kids that have had similar experiences, and our kids have all grown up to be well-rounded and compassionate individuals.

The other story I wanted to share about the effects of my conditions on my family took place on the medical floor of the hospital where I was working. My own lung disease, lymphangiomyomatosis, was under control, but we were still on edge about my prognosis as the condition is very rare. I go for yearly lung function tests, and while my breathing is fine for now we pray that I won't need that lung transplant down the road. At the time of this story I was still working full time as a surgical nurse and also on the medical units. One of my patients had a serious lung disease, could have been cancer but I don't remember for sure. He was a father in his late forties and had a daughter who was about nine years old. This patient, although very sick, was independent with all daily activities; I was only administering IV fluids, pain meds, and nebulizers to aid his breathing. He was doing the rest on his own. Within a matter of eight hours he took a turn for the worse, and when I arrived for my shift the next day he was bedbound and unresponsive. I had to call in his family to update them on his status. During my twelve-hour shift, his body was shutting down and he was no longer responding to treatment. We told the wife and daughter to say their goodbyes.

As a nurse, we see this scenario more than we care to mention; it comes with the job, and we handle it. But this time it was different for me. The scared little girl slowly walked over to her daddy to say goodbye, and I lost it. I couldn't hold back the tears. I had to excuse myself from the patient's room and gain my composure. All I could see was my own son Ben, who was the same age as the little girl, having to say good bye to me as I was dying on that hospital bed because of a serious lung disease. It was a reality I hope my family never has to face.

When I was reading the responses to the survey I sent out, I could see myself in many of the answers. The respondents were mostly women in their late twenties or early thirties experiencing symptoms of pain, weakness, and fatigue. Many of them were diagnosed with autoimmune diseases such as lupus, Sjogrens, Renaud's, diabetes, eczema, rheumatoid arthritis, osteoarthritis, Hashimoto's, and many others. They took anywhere from two to five prescribed medications daily, along with other supplements, but were willing to look into alternatives. Medical marijuana is still very new; not many had tried it besides me.

Most of the patients either had to change jobs to accommodate their chronic illness or, sadly, had to quit altogether and go on disability. Having experienced the latter myself, I know how devastating that can be. Letting go of my nursing career was heartbreaking, but I see now that it was the right decision for me and my family. I wish I had been easier on myself at the beginning, I would have saved myself a lot of heart ache. I thought I hadn't tried hard enough, but in truth I was trying too hard.

Another interesting fact reported was that swimming was a common source of exercise, which makes sense as it puts the least amount of stress on the joints as compared to other types of exercise. Walking was also another favorite.

Isolation and loneliness was another common factor for the people taking this survey. Many of the patients found that being part of group or organization that supports people with chronic illness, pain, and disabilities was extremely helpful. Knowing there are other people like you with similar issues that share a common goal—living with a better quality of life—is comforting and encouraging. I couldn't find a group in town when I was first diagnosed with systemic lupus, so I cofounded one with my dear friend Renuka. Our core group has been together for over thirteen years now. We no longer meet on a monthly basis to get an update on the latest happenings in the world of lupus, but we do make sure to have our spring brunch, summer picnic, and of course our annual Christmas Party. We put together fundraisers—usually a walk or pub night—and have fun together at the Annual Lupus Gala. Our group has brought in donations of over $150,000.00 to date. At one time I was also on the Lupus Canada Fund Development Board, but my health has gotten worse over the years and forced me to step back as the lead for fundraising. When we are meeting to catch up, we don't always talk about our illnesses. In fact, we usually look at photos and talk about our families, kids, and husbands, and occasionally we exchange information about treatments and medications or remember those we have lost to lupus complications.

Being part of group or organization becomes a culture that speaks its own language and has its own values and sense of purpose. I highly recommend looking into this type of support in your own community. I truly don't know I would have survived the first few years after my lupus without their love and support. Thank you to the members of the Surrey Lupus Group, the BC Lupus Society, and to Lupus Canada.

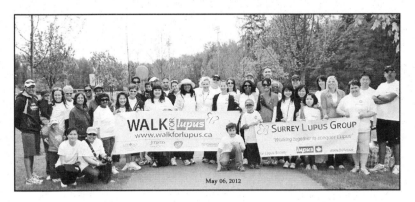

May 06, 2012

Journal reflection: When was the last time you talked to your loved ones about your lifestyle and any changes that need to be made?

_____

_____

_____

_____

Chapter 7

Screw you, I'm going to Nursing School!

I've always been driven and "stubborn," or so I'm told. I prefer to call myself determined. I wanted to make a difference in this world and I knew I had something special to offer. The next stage in my life would be difficult and scary, but I decided life was not worth waiting around for. I had to go out and get it. I needed to serve and help people.

A little while after my lupus diagnosis and my mild stroke, my mom and older sister were diagnosed with cancer within six months of each other; my mom with cervical cancer, and my sister with kidney cancer. When I was sitting in my mom's hospital room while she was recovering from the surgery to remove her tumour, I discovered that I felt at ease with all the equipment. I also had an inexplicable feeling that I could easily fit into this type of atmosphere. I watched as the nurse came and went with medications, IV bags, and needles to help patients feel better. I could do this. I'd already worked in Emergency Response, so how hard could it be?

Within a few weeks, I contacted a continuing education organization and registered to complete Biology 12, something I hadn't bothered taking in high school. At the time I was only experiencing some fatigue and mild aches from my chronic illnesses, so I figured I was good to get started on my next career path. I began my nursing courses in the fall of 2008 at the age of thirty-eight. I was one of the oldest people in my nursing class, which made me feel like mother hen to some of my classmates, but I did it. Age is only a number, and it's never too late to explore a new path. I remember thinking I was old at this time; now, I'm heading fast towards fifty. Apparently fifty is the new thirty though, so there!

What doesn't kill you still beats the crap out of you

The same week I started nursing school, I learned that my dear childhood friend Debi had suddenly passed away due to unforeseen circumstances during her battle with cancer. This news rocked me to my core. We had shared a wonderful friendship that spanned over twenty years. Our children played together as we'd share our health struggles. We'd compare notes about relationships and how illness impacted our lives and those of our families. She was one of the only friends I had that I could relate to, and I looked to her for inspiration and support. It was a very special friendship; we lifted each other up in ways that others could not. And now she was gone. Her two small children would have no mother. Her family was devastated. Her funeral was one of the most difficult services I had ever been to, and I sought solace in others whom had known her as well. It was such a huge loss of human life; she had a kind, beautiful, irreplaceable heart.

I still feel her loss to this day. I'm reminded of her whenever I hear certain songs on the radio. I remember us as kids, dressing up and pretending we were the lead singers for ABBA. Dancing Queen was our favourite song. We'd crank up the record in her basement and dance like nobody was watching, just us. I didn't have anyone I could relate to anymore. At that time I wasn't close to anyone else that had a chronic illness with a husband and kids to take care of. However, I knew that I needed to get my wits together and focus. She knew I was going into nursing school, so I decided I would do her proud. And I did.

About a month after she passed, I started having issues with kidney stones again. I went for an ultrasound to locate where the stone was as I kept getting bladder infections, which can be an indicator of a blocked kidney. The results were not what we expected. By accident, they had found a bunch of masses in both lungs during the kidney scan. After more testing, the specialist told me it was a very rare disease called lymphangiomyomatosis. These are small, sac-like cysts that grow inside the lungs and take up space. I would possibly need a lung transplant in the future, depending on how much the disease progresses.

My Respirologist sent me for pulmonary lung function tests every six months to evaluate my lung capacity and my oxygen exchange. At this point, the doctor suggested that because my medical condition was complicated, I should consider quitting nursing school and focusing on getting better.

Well then, they didn't know me very well, did they?

I ended up having three different procedures to prevent the kidney infection from getting worse. They were unable to operate to remove the stones until the infection was under control, so instead they inserted a stent through the urethra, up through the bladder, through the ureter and into the kidney to stop the stone from blocking the base of the kidney. A few weeks later, the stent somehow became infected and I was going septic. My blood pressure tanked at school and I was close to losing consciousness. My nursing instructor called my husband at work and explained the situation, so François picked me up and took my back to the hospital.

After a few complications, they were able to remove the stent and do a smash-and-grab to remove the stone; this procedure is called a cystoscopy. At this point they were finally able to remove the pieces of the broken stone from my kidney. I only missed one day of school that semester and wrote all my finals on morphine. My lowest mark was 92%; I guess I was so high on the pain meds that my test anxiety went away!

Just before my final semester, my mother was hospitalized a few times with Congestive Heart Failure. The worst part about being a nursing student is that you have all this new medical information, but you don't have the years of experience as a professional nurse to give you the calmness you need when a loved one is ill. My mother lived up in Shuswap, which is about five hours away by car, and would be undergoing a procedure where they would stop her heart and reset it. I had already started my acute care practicum, so if I left to be with her I'd fail the entire semester and miss graduating on time.

It was a difficult to decision to make, but my mom was very understanding and encouraged me to complete my practicum. She knew how hard I had worked so far and didn't want me to jeopardise my career. Thankfully, the procedure went well, and she is now in her seventies and quite healthy.

I completed nursing school, graduating with honours at the top of my class, and earned myself a job in a local hospital surgical unit where I did my acute care practicum. In our surgical unit, we mostly received patients from the ER for emergency surgeries; other patients would come via another unit with in the hospital or as transfer from another hospital. As a surgical nurse we had specific training that made us desirable to other units. Not only did we know how to respond to patients coming out of anesthetic, we also had experience in a lot of wound care as we were constantly checking and changing surgical wound sites. We also worked very closely with an interdisciplinary team of Occupational therapists, Physiotherapists, Respiratory Therapists, and Oncology, and of course the surgeons. As a result, we would frequently get called on to work in other areas.

The short-stay surgical patients were the best; they had to be mentally stable and independent as they shared a unit with the children. I hadn't taken special pediatric training yet, so I was only allowed to assist with the young patients. It broke my heart to see those kids away from home, scared and some without their parents. I was so grateful neither of our boys had ever been sick with anything dangerous other than the flu, and that our youngest did not show any signs of inheriting my lupus. My colleagues that worked in pediatrics were awesome, and I learned a lot from them.

I was lucky to have access to some amazing mentors in the form of other nurses who possessed many years of expertise in surgical nursing. We had the responsibility of ensuring the patients had stable vital signs, keeping on top of their pain control, and helping them remain as independent as possible in order to prepare them for going home. Of course, there was the odd patient that would never go home. We would then become palliative nurses and give comfort care, not only to patients but also to the families saying their last goodbyes to a loved one. That role I will always cherish and hold in my heart; it was a privilege to be there for those patients, holding their hand as they took their last breath. This experience also helped me understand how important my time is here on earth, and how grateful I am for what I have.

One shift, I was scheduled to work on one of the medical floors at the hospital and was partnered up with a nurse I hadn't yet worked with. We caught up on what happened with our patients the shift before, checking their charts for any doctor's orders that were new or discontinued and for any allergies or behaviours we needed to be aware of. Then we made sure we knew what meds they were taking, any diagnostic tests they may have had and any other specific treatments we'd be giving them, and how to best proceed with their care. Finally, we introduced of ourselves to each patient as we made our morning rounds.

About two to three hours later, I'd met all my patients and my partner and I were determining our break times for the next twelve hours. Suddenly, I felt something was off. I hadn't felt right all morning, and now I was feeling increasingly dizzy, lightheaded, and disoriented—not exactly the shape you want to be in when you're taking care of patients! I wasn't about to tell my new partner that I had medical issues of my own, though, as it wasn't anyone else's business unless I was putting myself, my partner, or my patients in danger. The next thing I knew, I woke up face down in a patient's room while my partner was calling for help. Apparently I'd bent down to empty a catheter bag and passed out. Before I could figure out what was going on, my charge nurse and my partner were on either side of me, holding me up by the shoulder and taking me to an empty treatment room. Embarrassed, I kept apologizing and trying to breathe but couldn't find the air. I could feel the room spin. When they took my blood pressure it was way too low, which was most likely the reason that I fainted.

My charge nurse called my husband to let him know what had happened, so he made his way to the hospital. Thank goodness I'd worked with her before and she knew my strong work ethic, so she knew this was something serious. She looked straight at me and demanded I tell her what was going on. Disoriented, I let my secret slip out and told her, aside from my lupus, I had also recently been diagnosed with left ventricular hypertrophy. Basically, the lupus was putting stress on my heart and causing it to work harder and become enlarged. I was on a new medication to try and stabilize my blood pressure, and clearly the medication was causing me to have orthostatic hypotension, meaning that every time I stood up too fast my blood pressure would bottom out and I'd pass out.

You can't be a nurse and be passing out at the same time. It's one or the other, not both. I was done for today. My charge nurse was a compassionate, although a bit ticked that I hadn't told anyone.

Becoming a nursing instructor

I took a short leave of absence to get my heart issue under control. During my absence, I received a call from one of my mentors, Anne. She had been one of my nursing instructors when I was a student and had left and incredible impression on me; I would be happy if I could be half the nurse that she was. Anne met me for coffee and invited me to apply for a teaching position as a Nursing Instructor. She felt I'd be a good fit because I'd already taught First Aid and CPR for so many years, and because I had been one of her favourite students, of course!

I started off working with the Coordinator of the Nursing program at the college in order to get familiar with the program and as the lab assistant instructor for Anne. I couldn't believe it, this was so cool. I was teaching nursing, and with the amazing Anne to boot! Wow!

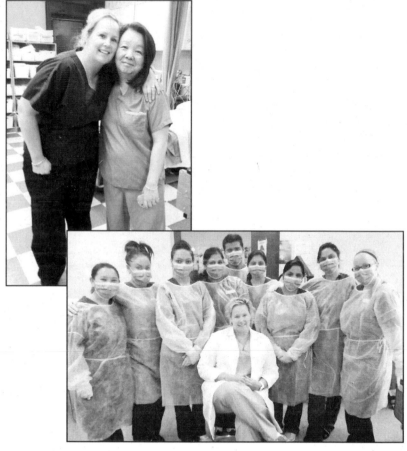

My first class was both exciting and nerve-racking, although Anne said I was a natural and fit right in. I eventually had my own group of students and taught theory for nursing communication, working with long-term care patients, acute care, clinical lab, and after a while I took over for the program coordinator, helping place students on their practicum. The best part was that I was partners with a nurse whom I'd looked up to for years! How could I get so lucky? Anne and I are still great friends. She invites me to her classes as a guest to speak of my experiences as an acute care nurse and an experienced patient.

I started to wonder if maybe this is where I was meant to be all along; it felt so right. I could make just as much a difference in the world not by saving patients, but by teaching others how to save them.

At one point, the college decided to let all of their part-time staff go, me included. No one was happy about this, especially not the students. They were so upset they even wrote a letter of protest to the director of the college and signed a petition to keep me as their instructor. Unfortunately, nothing could be done; it wasn't personal, just business. On my last day, my students threw me a big party. On the cake, they wrote the same affirmation I had given them on their first day: "Start where you are, use what you've got, do what you can." It was a quote I borrowed from tennis legend Arthur Ashe. I felt so blessed. I had learned so much from my students—they made me a better teacher and a better nurse.

After the bittersweet departure from the college, I went back to working at the hospital and started picking up extra shifts. By then my cardiologist had resolved my blood pressure issues. The director from another college called me not long after and offered me the position of lead instructor of their Health Care Assistant Program. I was thrilled at the idea of teaching again, so I started right away. The HCA program was similar to teaching the nursing program but with a different scope of practice—no IV, no given medication, and much less intense. It was going to be less stressful, or so I thought.

Soon after, I was offered the Regional Coordinator position as the current occupant was leaving. I hadn't applied for it, nor was I looking for anything above and beyond teaching, but a regional position would come with a larger paycheck, and with it larger and more complicated responsibilities. I was ultimately responsible for nine campuses, ensuring their compliance with the BC Care Aid Registry on every inch of that program, including instructor qualifications, lab layout and equipment specifications, writing and editing curriculum, exam policies, and clinical placement. It was challenging, exciting, fulfilling, and incredibly stressful. This is the position I held until my declining health forced me to retire.

Even though I can no longer work, my days of teaching are not over. Opportunities are starting to arise for me to share my story and help others in the same situation, one of them being this book. I may be down, but I'm not out!

Overcoming the obstacles

I've asked myself a few times, how did I possibly get through all the hardships and stress that I faced throughout these years, especially during nursing school? I can't say that there was any particular formula, but I'm sure it was a combination of a few things.

First of all, God was everywhere I needed Him to be in this crazy time of my life. I don't think I would have made it without His constant presence throughout these trials. My faith is one thing that I know for sure kept me going.

Next, having a support system in place is essential, although a bit tricky with chronic illnesses. Mine have come and gone over the years, which is normal as we grow and get older. But, there were some friends along the way that I felt had abandoned our friendship due my chronic illness and my inability to participate in the activities that I used to. I would have preferred to have been given the option of making the decision on my own as to whether or not I could take part, but often the decision was made for me and I just stopped getting invited. There is, however, a small but loyal group of friends that never gave up on me. They know who they are, and my family and I will forever be grateful for their support. This also includes our hockey family and our church family. Thank you for always being there for us!

One of the most important things you can do is to have some kind of plan, which is a bit of an ironic statement because making plans while living with chronic illness and pain is not always an easy thing to do. Plan on how you're going to get through work if you're not already on disability, or how you're going to manage your day-to-day activities.

Here is how we made our plan to overcome the obstacles:

1. Know **plans can change** at any given moment because of your illness, and be okay with this reality.
2. **Prepare for adaptations** in every plan you make; always have a plan B.
3. **Make it fun!** There's no point in trying to get something done if there's nothing fun about it.
4. Make **SMART goals** (Specific, Measurable, Attainable, Realistic, and Timely).
   a. Is the **goal specific to me** and geared for my pace?
   b. Can I **measure the achievement**, such as walking a certain distance that I haven't been able to do before?
   c. Am I **setting myself up for success or failure**? Is the possibility of success realistic for me ?

d. Can I do this **in a timely manner** that fits my life and schedule?

Another way of learning how to overcome obstacles or making changes for success is one of my old nursing tools called ADPIE:

- **Assess** your situation and recognize the signs & symptoms
- **Diagnose or determine** what the problems are
- **Plan** for overcoming or making your situation better, using SMART goals
- **Implement** your SMART goals, get your plans into motion
- **Evaluate** if your new adaptations have worked, if not go back and re-assess.

I borrowed this from the North American Nursing Diagnosis Association. We used to teach this formula to nursing students to use for making care plans for our patients, but there's no reason why you can't use it to help overcome your own challenges.

Journal reflection: How have you overcome obstacles in your life?

_____

_____

_____

_____

Chapter 8

Mental health and chronic pain

As I created this book, I originally avoided this chapter for fear of judgement. However, I felt compelled to write it as I know there will be someone out there going through the same scary process, experiencing a multitude of pain and losses. I write this in hopes that it will encourage either a patient or their family members to recognize that these struggles are real, and sometimes dark, but that joy and happiness is also possible.

I feel frozen in time when I think about all the stress I've had to cope with. Was I safe to be alone? Am I taking my pain medications when my pain is not that bad? Am I avoiding social or family events for fear of conversations I don't know how to have? I'm worried I'll see that look on their faces of either disbelief or pity, neither of which I want. It's just all too much.

Scientists believe stress can cause us to have ill health down the road. Some doctors use a test called The Holmes-Rahe

Stress Inventory, a forty-three-question test created in 1967 by psychiatrists Thomas Holmes and Richard Rahe, to determine how susceptible you might be to a stress-induced health breakdown after experiencing stressful events. I scored over 300 on the test, which indicates I'm mostly likely to be ill for the next two years! Breathe and be still, Leisa, breathe and be still. Meditation and prayer have really helped me improve my mental health; so did leaving my nursing career in exchange for getting my health back on track. Make sure that if you do take this test, you don't panic if you get a bad result. Instead, talk to your doctor about getting help with reducing your stress levels.

"Be still and know that I am God."
Psalm 46:10 (NIV)

∾

November 8, 2017

It's hard to stay within a deadline for writing a book when you have painful flare ups that prevent you from sitting down or writing for too long. This is one of those times. It is Autumn right now, which is when flare ups occur more frequently, triggered by the weather changing to cooler, damper temperatures here in Vancouver. It's also flu season. Writing this book is one of the hardest thing I've ever done in my life. It's scary. I'm afraid of judgement and of not finishing on time. Will it be good enough? Will it make sense? Most importantly, will it help someone? I persevere with the knowledge that I feel compelled to help at least one person with my story. I have approximately three months left to write before we go to the editing part of the creation of this book.

How do I write when I in so much pain? My husband gave me some encouraging words today. He offered the advice he gives himself when he works on a custom piece of art: take one step at a time. Even if it's only one paragraph, or one line, just do it. Then, at the end of the day, you can say, "I did it!" He was right, of course, but it's so easy to make excuses because of the physical pain. I'm hearing my own voice in my head as I encourage others with the same approach, "One step at a time." I'm also hearing echoes of my wonderful publisher Julie saying, "Be kind to yourself."

~

Here's a few tips on how to reduce your stress level an improve your mental health. First of all, **get up and breathe!** Take three to ten slow, deep breaths, in through your nose and out through your mouth. Oxygen flow helps with healing.

Move more. Exercise is so vital to our health. It's not easy when you're in constant pain, so start low and go slow. A short walk, even just to get groceries, counts as physical activity. It's also great stress buster! **Stretching every morning** helps me assess which parts of my body are going to be a problem and which ones are working well. Active stretching also increases circulation and body temperature, which allows for easier movement.

Have a shower! Not only does it make you feel better, it gets you clean. Routine hygiene is essential for maintaining skin integrity and prevents pressure ulcers if you're on bed rest or sitting for prolonged periods.

Eat something healthy. Breakfast is the most important meal of the day. Your body needs fuel! Make sure your nutrition is balanced and try to eat less sugar as it feeds infections and creates fat. On a similar note, make sure you're **drinking enough water**. Being well-hydrated helps with digestion, improves muscle function, protects your brain and joints, keeps skin healthy, maintains body temperature, keeps your bowels moving, and flushes out toxins.

Take your medication on time and keep your prescriptions up to date. This helps reduce stress when it comes time for a refill.

Meditation or prayer are both calming and grounding. Try using meditation and prayer apps with daily messages to keep your spirit strong. You can also try **listening to music**, which is healing to the soul. It also reduces stress and depression, aids sleep, and strengthens learning and memory.

Engage in an activity that involves other people. When I focus on the needs of others, it takes my mind off of my own issues. It also makes me feel good to know that I am helping someone else.

Last but not least, **have some fun!** Do something you enjoy or makes you laugh. Laughter is beneficial to your physical, emotional, and spiritual health.

When you're living with chronic pain, your mental health is intertwined with your physical health. They cannot be separated, so they must both be recognized. If you don't allow yourself the grace of healing and patience, there will almost always be an overwhelming feeling of not accomplishing anything and wasting your time.

Here's what has helped me cope.

You need to tell someone when these feelings of inadequacy take over. I don't always feel like expressing my feelings out loud; however, the alternative is that it stays inside and festers, allowing my very creative mind to manifest some crazy and unrealistic goals. There will be days, like the one I had yesterday, where you just sit on the couch in your pajamas and rest. The trick is to not have more than two of those days in a row as it can lead to a fixation on self-doubt, and then suddenly you're on your way to a pity party. Of course, if you have doctor's orders for bed rest, that is a whole separate issue. Just be clear about the reasons why you must do nothing today.

My sister shared with me a realization she had that had a huge impact on her when she came from California for a visit last spring. She stayed with us at our house so her and I could have some much-needed sister time. She said that she knew I was living with chronic pain, but she didn't realize how bad it was or how much it affected my everyday life until she saw it for herself. It made me realize that with invisible illnesses, unless I verbalize that I'm experiencing physical or emotional pain, no one will really know what I'm dealing with. However, there are several reasons why I tend not to speak up:

1. Maybe they won't believe me, because they said I don't look sick.
2. I'm still walking and talking, so it can't be that bad.
3. I didn't have to take that many pain killers today, so I shouldn't make too much fuss.
4. I'm a nurse, so I always know how to handle it
5. I'm tired of hearing it, so they must be too.
6. I've lost too many friendships already, I don't want to risk losing another.
7. I don't want people to worry, especially my parents and my kids.
8. I know there is always someone way worse off than I am, so I shouldn't complain.
9. Maybe if I ignore the pain, it will go away.

10. I just want to be "normal" and not have pain and illness as my identity.

Having to live with chronic pain and illness forces you into a lifestyle you didn't want. It's a huge loss, especially if you were an athlete and an adrenaline seeker such as myself. One of the theories we teach to nursing students is the five stages of grief, developed by Elizabeth Kubler Ross. The stages are described as are denial, anger, bargaining, depression, and acceptance. You don't often progress linearly through these stages; you can end up circling back through the different stages in no particular order if we haven't been able to move forward and stop grieving. I use this theory as a measuring stick as to how I'm doing with my grief due to the losses I've experienced with my chronic illness.

What my friends and family may not know

Most people that know me see me as a happy, vibrant, energetic person. Those that know me well know that I have good days and bad days, just like everyone else. What might shock people to know, though, is that I've contemplated suicide. I didn't plan anything out or try to hurt myself; I was just stuck in a deep depression that lead me to be thinking the world might be better off if I wasn't here anymore. I thought it would be easier for everyone if I wasn't around, but I realized that this wasn't true. They'd be dealing with the great loss of a loving, caring, funny, courageous human being that is irreplaceable: ME.

I'm happy to say that I've recovered from that way of thinking and now recognize that we all have moments of deep sadness that can send our thoughts into a dark, unimaginable place. I'm sure there are many people that have had the same, if not similar, contemplation about "not being here." However, suicide does not solve the problem; it only complicates everything and leaves behind a tragedy and despair that can never be repaired. I have my faith in God to thank for this realization. I also have the blessing of having a wonderful, encouraging husband who sees me at my worst and knows when I've hit rock bottom. In addition, my parents have played an integral part in my recovery by being there whenever we needed them.

Let me explain why I use the word recovery to refer to getting healthier. Overcoming mental illness is a process, much like a recovery from and injury or an addiction. We must follow a proven course that will lead us into a better way of living, a better way of thinking, and a better way to move forward with all aspects of our health. I believe that unless we have our mind, body, and spirit in a positive state, then we are not healthy; we are simply living without illness. The very definition of wellbeing includes all three of these areas.

Another significant support for my mental health is my tribe. If you don't have a tribe, you need to get one! A tribe is a group of positive, forward-thinking, like-minded souls that lift you up. They not only help you get out of those dark spaces, but they also champion you to achieve above and beyond your own expectations.

I thank you all for bringing me back to myself. I'm forever grateful that I will always have your support!

Journal reflection: What can you do to take better care of your mental health?

_____

_____

_____

_____

Chapter 9

You don't look sick

We've all heard that aggravating statement: "You don't look sick, you must be feeling better!" Some days I *am* feeling better than usual, but it has nothing to do with my appearance. Ask anyone living with chronic pain and they will tell you trying to "look normal" takes way more effort than just lying on the couch in agony.

Even though it is hard to pretend that we are feeling okay, people with chronic illnesses may still choose to try and hide their conditions. We may do this because we want to protect our loved ones from the ugliness of our suffering, or because we are afraid of losing a job or other opportunities. Often, we're worried about being judged by friends, family, and colleagues. Some days, it's also easier to just say you're "fine" rather than explain all the complicated, gory details, and at the end of the day it's really no one else's business anyway.

We struggle with people judging us. We battle with our own inner dialogue of "am I really sick enough that I need to bother someone about it?" We ignore our symptoms because we are sure no one wants to hear about it for the millionth time this week. People avoid us because of how much pain we are in, or how difficult it was for us to get in and out of a chair, or how frustrated we get waking up every morning with yet another part of our body that refuses to cooperate. For our struggles to be brushed off because we don't outwardly look sick is absolutely infuriating.

One of the most difficult challenges of having an invisible chronic illness is having to convince people how sick you are. It hardly seems fair. There are already so many obstacles that we have to overcome each and every day; one of them should not have to be covering up our illness or pain to make other people feel more comfortable just because we don't "look" sick enough. I will never apologize for being true to who I am and how I am feeling in that moment. I can tell you, however, it sure takes an incredible amount of strength to NOT do something that we really want to so that we don't pay for it later. This is probably the most difficult but necessary responsibility we owe to ourselves and our loved ones around us.

I can't tell you how many times I've been glared at while parking in a handicapped spot, and it's an awful feeling to have people look at you like your cheating the system. Believe me, if I didn't have to be using a handicapped spot, I wouldn't! There are lots of days when I don't use it, even if it's the best parking spot on the lot, because I don't need it that day and someone else may need it more.

I worked in Therapeutic Recreation for nine years, and it would anger me when I brought a wheelchair-bound client to the pool and found an able-bodied person idling in a designated parking spot, waiting to pick someone up. I had many a heated conversation with a few thoughtless people about how they were "only going to be five minutes." For example, I once had to go to a medical appointment and there was no parking left. My hip was very painful that day and I had trouble walking, but I had to take the only available spot, which was down the street at a park. When I arrived at my doctor's office parking lot, I noticed a lady parked and waiting in the handicapped spot. I tapped on her window and politely stated that she had forgotten her disability window pass. She blatantly stated she wasn't handicapped, she was just waiting for her husband and this was the only spot available. I pulled out my disability parking pass from my purse and told her it's not available to you unless you have a permit, and that I had been forced to limp all the way down the street with my bad hip because of her. She sheepishly nodded and rolled up her window. Unbelievable! This person's ignorance just made me so angry. The fact that I have to face the consequences of living with chronic pain is frustrating all by itself; I shouldn't have to explain my situation to careless people as well.

What I'd like for people to know is that being on disability does not mean that we're on vacation! Most of us would much rather go back to work and be "normal" again, earning a paycheck and having the respect and comradery of our colleagues. I loved my nursing career, and I miss it terribly every day. I was forty-six when I had to retire because of the serious health complications I faced with my systemic lupus, osteoarthrosis, sciatica, and fibromyalgia. I feel like I still have so much to offer, but I know that being home and taking care of myself was the right decision for me and my family. I can be replaced at work, but I can never be replaced at home.

This doesn't mean that I'm out lounging in the sun on the

beach or shopping though. Trying to be healthy with multiple chronic illnesses is a very lonely and isolating full-time job. Depression has hit me harder since I've had to go on disability; thankfully, there are people in my life that help me manage. It isn't easy asking for help, but it's worth letting people who care about you at least give it a shot. You will have to be honest and tell them what you need. You'll find out very quickly who's genuinely concerned and who's only being polite. Keep the people who truly care for you close, and make sure you tell them how much you appreciate their offer.

Behind the scenes

Most healthy people can just pop out of bed, hop into the shower, quickly get dressed, have breakfast, and get moving for the day in the span of an hours' time. For someone living with multiple chronic illness like myself, this is definitely not the case. To give you an idea of what living with a chronic illness can be like, I'm going to share some of the challenges I face during my day that a healthy person wouldn't even have to think about.

My preparation for the day actually starts the night before. I prepare my clothing for the next day, especially if I know I'm meeting someone or have an appointment to go to. This will save me time in the morning if my pain limits my mobility. I also try to have my shower before I go to bed rather than taking one in the morning; showers take a lot of energy, so they work best if I can lay down right afterwards.

Getting out of bed can be challenging. The amount of effort it takes really depends on how much I exerted myself the day before and how well I slept. On a good day, it takes me about thirty minutes to crawl out of bed; on a bad day, I require a longer transition time and some assistance. I log-roll to get to the edge of the bed and spend some time some re-positioning and stretching my hips and spine to prepare for getting up. When I'm ready, I sit up, and then I wait. Breathe. Then try to stand and see how stable my legs, hips, back, and neck are feeling and whether they are going to cooperate. Once I'm up, I head straight for my CBD oil; this is medical marijuana that I take every morning to help with pain and inflammation. Some days I have François bring me a heating pad for my back, and I'll rest with this for a good twenty to thirty minutes. I try to get dressed; this can take a good ten to fifteen minutes unaided, although some days the pyjamas don't come off at all. We're already an hour and half in and I haven't even made it down the stairs yet!

Now that I'm home all the time, my day is determined first by any medical appointments I may have. On a regular bi-weekly basis I see my RMT and my Chiropractor. I see my GP on a monthly basis. Every few months I see my Rheumatologist and any other specialists. Some days I may need to go for x-rays, blood work, urine analysis, MRI, CT scans, or heart monitoring. Currently, I'm an outpatient for the Pain Clinic. There I see a Doctor for cortisone injections for both of my hips and spinal injections to have the peripheral nerves frozen and cauterized. Both procedures are painful, and I'm out of commission for up to three days afterwards. They also have a Physiotherapist and a Social worker that I will see from time to time for counselling and exercise.

If my pain is not under control or I have limited mobility, I'm at home for the day on the couch with heat, ice, pain meds and my favorite blanket, possibly with chocolate nearby. I try not to stay in bed, it's too depressing.

If I'm not going to a medical appointment and my pain

is under control, I do restorative yoga twice a week with my amazing yoga instructor, Karen Pledger. She has designed her class specifically so I can be there in the calm and peacefulness; even on days when I can't fully participate, she welcomes me to lie down and just be. On the other days she takes the time to do a private lesson in my home so if I require pain meds, I don't have to drive. I love her! Thank you Karen!

On good days when I am mobile and feeling okay, François takes me out for lunch or on walks with our dog to the beach or the forest. Being by the ocean and in the trees are my happy places, other than shopping of course! I sometimes meet my Mom or a friend for coffee, while other days I'm happy to just be close to home puttering in the garden, reading a good book, or even writing one!

Dinner is another challenge as my activity level tends to slow down towards midday. This means I have to prepare meals in advance, usually with some assistance. François has some great crockpot recipes, which are really helpful for me because they can be started early in the day. If I don't start the meal prep early enough, we end up getting takeout or eating leftovers. After dinner, I have to prep for the next day and it all starts over again. However, most days my body has already shut down by then and meals get put on the backburner—pun intended!

Another good perspective on what it's like to like with a chronic illness is a theory called "The spoon theory" (available at www.butyoudontlooksick.com), created by another lupus patient, Christine Miserandino. It's basically a story of a day in life of a lupus patient. I like to describe it like an energy bank or ATM, but she uses spoons to demonstrate her point. Every decision and task you make will cost you a spoon. You must plan out every single step for your day and understand that at any given time you can run out of energy, or "spoons" as Christine calls it. People who are healthy take for granted simple everyday things like getting out of bed, getting dressed, sitting at a desk, cooking, or cleaning. For someone with a chronic illness, something as simple as getting in and out of a car may use up a "spoon" and prevent you from doing something else later in the day.

I used to struggle with feeling inadequate as a wife and mother because I couldn't do what I felt like I should be doing. Thankfully, I have learned to let go of these feelings. I'm blessed with the fact that my wonderful boys have become understanding about my limitations after witnessing firsthand my decline in activity. I used the word "become" because in the early years, they weren't able to comprehend the challenges I faced. We had to learn together and adapt. They now know that I do the best I can, and they are quick to remind me if I'm doing too much. Unfortunately, unless you live with someone with chronic illness, it's difficult to imagine what struggles they face. Hopefully, though, this chapter has given you a little more insight.

It's extremely challenging to live with someone with chronic illness, especially when that person has multiple chronic illnesses and daily pain. It's all about communication, love, patience, kindness, and treating each other and yourself with respect. Without those elements present, the stress of an unbalanced environment can cause your illness to progress and leave your household in danger of falling apart.

Journal reflection: What do you do to show self-love?

_____

_____

_____

_____

Chapter 10

The digestive system and other shitty things—a poop story

When I was a nursing instructor, I taught all the body systems among other nursing and health care programs. One of my favourites was the digestive system, because it tells us so much about our bodies—what we put in, what gets used, what doesn't get used, and how foods, minerals, and medications metabolize. What we don't need gets pooped out. By looking at the size, shape, consistency, and frequency of a person's bowel movements, you can learn so much about their health. I decided that it is not just a shitty topic, it is my favourite shitty topic, and I ended up being known around campus for my poop talk!

When I worked as a surgical nurse, it was imperative to always keeping an eye on my patient's bowel movements; this was part of the standard treatment and protocol for recovery after surgery. If a patient wanted to go home, the fastest way to get there was to have a good bowel movement on your own. It needed to be of the right colour, shape, size, and consistency as well. Things like immobility, the wrong diet, and medication can take away from consistent bowel movements, so we need to make efforts to ensure our bowels keep moving. Although meant for a hospital setting, this bowel protocol is also recommended for at home.

Fluids are essential, as long as the Doctor approves, as water and other clear fluids—such as apple or cranberry juice, tea or black coffee, chicken or beef broth, ginger ale, and Jell-O—help keep the stool from becoming too hard to pass and prevent blockages in the bowels. Being mobile, as much as you are allowed to, is encouraged as well. Movement increases our peristalsis, the wave-like muscle contractions that move food through our system, which helps keep our internal organs healthy and our digestive system moving.

Medications, especial opioids, can cause constipation and block up your bowels. In this case, there are some options. Taking pain meds that are not opioids may not be as effective for treating pain, but they won't cause constipation either. If you do need to take opioid medications, make sure you are drinking lots of clear fluids to counteract the constipation that comes with them. Avoid full fluids such as milk and yogurt, which can make constipation worse. You may also consider taking a stool softener before bed or in the morning if needed; they help soften the stool to help it pass.

If a stool softener is not effective, you may consider taking a laxative. These are a more active medication that pushes the stool out much faster, sometimes causing diarrhea if you're not careful. It's important to mention that laxatives can be detrimental to your natural digestive system; if taken frequently, your bowels may become dependent on the laxative and you may not be able to produce a stool on your own. The best practice to keep your bowels moving is for you to keep active and drinks lots of water.

Eating more fibre can help keep your digestive system moving, but beware of adding fibre after you're already constipated. This is a common mistake I would see over and over again in the hospital. If you're already blocked up, adding fibre simply creates more bulk, which can then become a blockage and send you to the emergency room. If you're having problems with constipation, speak to your family doctor and discuss the best solution for you and your situation. Don't stop taking any medication without advice from your doctor.

I have a funny story about my own digestive system under attack, which occurred when I was the Regional Coordinator for Vancouver Career College and CDI for their Health Care Assistant Program. My teaching days were fewer than I would have liked and I was spending more time in my office in front of the computer, editing curriculum or on the phone with one of the nine campuses I was responsible for. So, when one of my campus Directors called me in a panic because the instructor of a new group of nursing students had called in sick, I jumped at the chance to fill in and go teach. I knew they were desperate for someone to cover as I was usually their last resort, and I was happy to get out of my office and spend a day or two doing what I loved.

My digestive system had been flaring up for a few weeks up to this point. I'd been blocked up and unable to poop for several days, so I'd taken a stool softener the night before to get things moving, if you will. Unfortunately, I didn't realize at the time that the softeners I'd taken had a laxative included. As I mentioned earlier, a stool softener only softens your poop in order to encourage it to come out easier. A laxative on the other hand not only softens the poop, it also helps speed up the rate at which it comes out. In my case, it came out URGENTLY!

So, back to my story. I've taken what I thought was just stool softener the night before. I may have even taken two! I began my drive to the campus, which takes approximately forty-five minutes depending on traffic, sipping my travel mug of coffee along the way. I was about three-quarters of the way there when my stomach started to complain. You know that familiar grumble; the one that tells you that you'd better get to where you're going fast or there's going to be a problem. I started to sweat as the grumbling and cramping became a bit more frequent. I'm in full-blown—and I literally mean literally full-blown—atomic farting mode now! I open the window, struggling for fresh air. As I started to wonder what I ate, it suddenly hit me. Oh shit! The stool softener/laxative, combined with the coffee, was creating an internal explosive nuclear weapon that was looking for an exit. I'm now in panic mode, clenching and shaking as I desperately searched for a gas station. Unfortunately, I was stuck in traffic and couldn't turn off anywhere. Oh my gosh, what am I to do?

The farts were now getting questionable and the cramps were excruciating. I was getting closer to my destination, but I knew I wasn't going to make it. Thankfully, at this point I spotted a Tim Horton's just around the corner. Just in time! I pulled in the parking lot and left everything in the car, including my purse and wallet, and I ran with my cheeks clenched, shoving people out of the way and yelling "excuse me!" as I prayed to the almighty above that the bathroom was free. It was. As I slammed and locked the door, poop was escaping down my leg and onto the floor. At last I finally get to the toilet and my body literally explodes with the remainder of what's left in my sigmoid colon. I carefully step out of my underwear and pants and wonder what I should do. How can I go teach a class of nursing students with no pants on? Wait, how do I get out of the Tim Hortons with no pants?

I tried to calm down and told myself to use my critical thinking and come up with a plan. I knew the underwear was a write-off; I wasn't even going to try and save them. The pants weren't too bad, so I washed what I could and stood butt-naked in the Tim Hortons bathroom, drying my pants under the air dryer. Thankfully it wasn't just paper towel! Once the pants were dry, I rinsed them a second time and then went back to the air dryer. My quick thinking worked; I now had semi-clean pants. I went commando and left the Tim Hortons bathroom, feeling sorry for the employee that would discover the nuclear disaster in the bathroom garbage. Miraculously, I made it to class on time with none the wiser to my situation. After this event, I started keeping an extra pair of underwear in the glove compartment just in case; these came in handy when this happened again later that month! True story!

The purpose of sharing this story is to demonstrate the many complications of living with systemic lupus. Our autoimmune systems can attack any organ at any time, and this time my digestive system was under attack. We have to be very aware of our diet as certain foods can complicate our digestive system. There is no one diet that works for everyone; it's very individual and usually worked out by trial and error. I have to take caution with foods that cause inflammation, such as dairy (including the cream I use in my coffee every morning). I also made the mistake of making it worse by using the wrong medication. Bad nurse! By paying attention to our bowels, though, we can get a great picture of our overall health.

Journal reflection: How often to do you have bowel movements? Is it more or less than every 2-3 days?

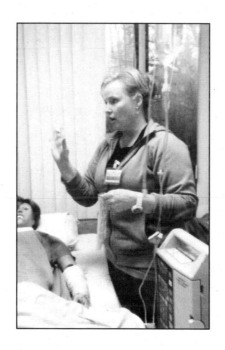

Chapter 11

Committing to change

November 13, 2015

An envelope arrived in the mail today; one of those ominous recycled government envelopes. My husband handed it to me, having already opened it by mistake.

Here it was, in black and white. "The Canadian Pension Plan for Disability has acknowledged receipt of your application and medical reports for receiving disability benefits." I couldn't breathe, and my eyes filled with tears of disbelief. What had I done? Am I really doing this? Did I give up too easy? The moment of panic gave way to tears of grief. It was done.

I had passed the first two of the three required criteria, the first being that I had contributed enough hours to CPP over my life and the second being that they received a signed medical report from my doctor. Phase three was the last step. My application had to pass through the government's medical adjudicator to determine if I was capable of returning to work. The written document was brief but to the point; they would decide if what I had was ever going to get better or not, and I should expect to hear their decision in a window of six to eight weeks' time.

Our youngest son, Ben, asked my husband what was wrong. Why was Maman crying? My husband carefully explained it in a way that a thirteen-year-old hockey fanatic could understand. "Imagine you get a letter in the mail that says you are no longer allowed to play hockey ever again for the rest of your life. It doesn't matter how much you want to play or how good you are, you're never allowed to play again." Our son went upstairs to avoid seeing me cry while my husband took me in his arms to comfort me. I thought the wound from this emotional trauma had healed a few weeks ago. Now it was ripped open like a day two post-operative surgical site, fresh and painful.

The next few days I kept finding myself back on that damned emotional rollercoaster I thought I'd already gotten off of. I'd find myself thinking that I couldn't do this again. I don't want to feel helpless and vulnerable anymore. I just want this grieving to stop. I want to call Dr. Kubler-Ross, the scholar who came up with the five stages of grief, and scream "go to hell!" into the phone. I thought I was at the acceptance stage, but that was a crock of shit! I'm back a stage three again! Or is it stage four? I don't know, I'm so confused and pissed off. Perfect, now I'm back and stage two!

～

January 11, 2016

Another government envelope arrived to tell me that my application for disability had been denied. I was shocked! Did they not read my letter and medical files properly? The next step was to fight back and appeal the decision. Below is the letter I have written and sent to them; now, we wait. It will be another three months before a final decision is made.

Dr. xxxx xxxx   *January 11, 2016*
Medical Adjudicator
Service Canada

This letter shall serve as my appeal for CPP Disability that was denied Dec 17, 2015. I received this notice on Dec 23, 2015. I implore you to reconsider your decision.

Gainful employment is not going to be determined by whether or not I have back surgery. All the other debilitating limitations I have are preventing me from working. The new lumbar and neck issues have just made the list of complications longer and should not be used solely to decide my limitations.

I have been struggling with systemic lupus for over ten years, along with fibromyalgia, osteoarthritis, lymphangiomyomatosis, Sjogrens, Reynaud's, nerve damage, asthma, and migraines. As you are aware these are incurable diseases that leave me debilitated on a regular basis. These conditions are only made tolerable with analgesics, muscle relaxants, anti-inflammatories, and narcotics, but will be indefinite in duration. These disabilities have left me unable to work and drive as determined by my family doctor, Dr. XXXX, as well as my lupus specialist, Dr. XXXXXX. More recently, the pain in my lumbar spine, hip damage, and neck deterioration have complicated matters.

My doctors and I were all shocked to learn that I did not meet the CPP Disability medical requirements. It is difficult to understand the decision that I do not suffer severe pain with the above-mentioned joint, muscle, and tissue diseases. I can only sit or stand for short periods of time which would prevent me from any kind of work, not just as a Nurse Educator.

Agreed, there is a new medication for nerve pain that has been somewhat helpful; however, it still does not allow me to function enough to drive or work on some days. This type of pain is completely unpredictable. Nerve medication causes nausea, light-headedness, confusion, disorientation, and difficulties with balance. The unfortunate part of living with multiple chronic illnesses is that the medication, although helpful, also comes with side effects that can be worse than the original symptoms, making it more difficult to function on a daily basis.

The statement that the "connective tissue disease is not currently active" does not stop the pain and debilitating limitations caused by all the other diseases. It simply means that the ANA blood work for the lupus was not at high range at the time of the last visit. These numbers change regularly and does in no way indicate that there is no inflammation process occurring in the joints or elsewhere in the body.

The painful facet joint injections can only be given every three months per area so I may maintain mobility. One month it's shoulders, then elbows, then knees, then hips. This is not a new treatment; I have been receiving these for a few years now and the benefits are only temporary. Physiotherapy is not a new treatment for me either, it is just being applied to a new area on my body. I've been using alternative therapies for years, including chiropractic care, registered massage therapy, connective tissue therapy, ultrasound, hydrotherapy, and acupuncture. They are for maintenance and do not cure the diseases. Sometimes they work; sometimes, they only trigger the inflammation.

The MRI is quite evident and clearly explains the damage in the lumbar area. I am unclear as to why this is even in question. The only question at this point is how they are going to try and give me some kind of relief. There is no request for a second opinion. However, I am on a wait list to see the neurosurgeon to decide if I should have back surgery or not. The diagnosis itself is not being disputed. His decision won't change my outcome for my employment status. I can't be expected to function on narcotic or nerve pain medication 24/7. It is not realistic and is very damaging to the liver, not to mention that it's dangerous and illegal to operate a vehicle when on these medications. Beyond the lumbar radiculopathy, all the other complications of the joint damage and other conditions are debilitating enough on their own.

Please reconsider your decision. Giving up my nursing licence was not an easy decision for me to make; in fact, it was one of the most difficult things I have ever had to do. I am only forty-six years old, but my health has continually deteriorated over the years and it is time to stop pushing my body beyond what it can handle. I have tried scaling back to part-time and then even working from home, which has only proven that when at home I can lie down or take stronger medication with a sedative as a side effect, which prevents me from working anyway.

The quality of life that everyone deserves to have should not come at the cost of family. I should not have to choose between forcing myself to suffer for hours at a time, and then coming home and having to go straight to bed from pain and exhaustion. This has been extremely difficult for my family to watch me go from working Search and Rescue, Disaster Response, and Surgical Nurse; to being a Nurse Educator/ Regional Coordinator; to doing nothing. I played fast ball for twenty-six years, soccer for sixteen years, hiked, skied, and ran until up until my diagnosis in 2005. They have watched me slow down significantly and sadly as I lose a part of myself with every new diagnosis and every activity I miss out on.

Thank you for your time and consideration,
Leisa Cadotte

∼

April, 2015

Asked Ben when he got home from school today, did he feel bad that I was often sick or in too much pain to be able to do things with him? Or, did his friends ever ask him why his mom was always in her pyjamas when they come over? Or, did he feel like I didn't give him enough attention, and did I leave him alone too much to fend for himself? He very clearly stated, "No." Did he want me to stay at home full time, again a resounding "no." He thought it was good for me to be out the house so he could have a break from having me around, and that the only thing that bothered him was that I missed too many of his hockey games. Ouch! I really thought he saw how much effort I was putting into being there. However, I need to remind myself that he's only fourteen, and I did ask!

A few months' later, just days after Ben's fifteenth birthday, he stated that he didn't know how I could live with so much pain every day. He said he was sad for me. Then, he wanted to know if we had any snacks.

~

March 29, 2016

Today was my second fluoroscopy injection in two weeks on my SI joints. I've given a brief outline to explain where in the body this takes place, as described by medical author Catherine Burt Driver, MD:

The sacroiliac (SI) joints are formed by the connection of the sacrum and the right and left iliac bones. The sacrum is the triangular-shaped bone in the lower portion of the spine, below the lumbar spine. The iliac bones are the two large bones that make up the pelvis. As a result, the SI joints connect the spine to the pelvis. The sacrum and the iliac bones (ileum) are held together by a collection of strong ligaments. These joints need to support the entire weight of the upper body when we are erect, which places a large amount of stress across them. This can lead to wearing of the cartilage of the SI joints and arthritis.

Average age of patients that have sacroiliac problems are over fifty-five. I'm forty-six. This is not unheard of in my age group, though, as we know arthritis does not discriminate.

The sun was beautiful, so when I got home decided to try walk with my cane to the mail box. Remember, I've just had fluoroscopy procedure two hours prior, so I have a frozen ass, quad, and hamstring and my balance was off. I'd also taken a few T3s for good measure. It took me a good fifteen minutes to get there and back; usually, it only takes about in two to three minutes. As I was returning to my house I noticed the signs we have placed in our complex due to the fact there are often children playing outside. The sign said "slow." *No shit,*

I thought to myself, *I'm going slowly*. But hey, at least I'm still mobile and independent! This will be the last of my injections for a while as we feel the risk outweighs the benefits.

~

April, 2016

I received the call from the government-appointed medical adjudicator on April first; funny that it was April Fool's Day! It was also the same day my dear friend Tammy was laid to rest. I was unable to go to the funeral as I was overcome, suffering with severe anxiety over my bodyweight and illness. I knew there would be friends from high school there, and they all were in great shape and had amazing careers. I didn't want to have to explain why I was walking with a cane, so overweight, and no longer working. I was literally paralyzed by fear and couldn't leave the house.

The phone call came from a wonderful nurse who said she saw my appeal case for CPP disability as a no-brainer. It was clear to her that I wasn't getting better, nor would I if I continued to work. I needed to stay at home to try and get my health back.

There is no cure for most of the diseases I have, but I could at least rest when I needed and have the time to try and get better and spend time with my family. I'd already missed out on so much.

~

June 28, 2016

Feet are swollen badly again today. Something must be happening with my blood pressure and/or the medication. Then again, it could be kidney related. Fluids tend to flow with gravity and pool in the feet. Oh well, I'm going to aqua fit anyway with my cane, who I've named Hugo. He goes everywhere I want him too, even to the pool! I'm somewhat embarrassed as I approach the ladder and steps to get into the water. The class is for seniors and I'm only forty-six. I think the instructor is like ninety-something, but she can move a whole lot better than I can. The group sympathetically stares at me as I enter the water; some look away so I don't see the look of pity on their faces. This is my reality, but hey, me and Hugo, we got this!

I have been meeting up with some wonderful women entrepreneurs to meet and greet and also hear a few of them speak. They would share a bit of their story and how they got their business started. They did such a great job facilitating, I thought to myself that it was just like teaching to my healthcare and nursing students. I could do this no problem, I've been presenting for years! I approached the event coordinator and bravely told her I was ready to tell my story of overcoming living with multiple chronic illness and having to retire early. She was thrilled and added my name to list. I'm super excited!!

∼

June 29, 2016

Oh no, what have I done? I'm now fully freaking out! Why did I tell the organizer that I was ready to share my story?

Why did I tell her I could go on stage and present? I'm so not ready for this yet! The swelling in my feet has gone down. I'm sure its anxiety. No, no it's not. I'm losing my mind, it's just cardiac-related stuff.

Today that ugly familiar feeling of discouragement hovers over me about my bodyweight staying the same and not going in direction I want it to. I was being careful—maybe its water weight? There's enough fluid in both ankles to float a frigging submarine! Then again, it could very well be hormones. Lord knows. I'm disgusted with myself. [I would later learn that the swelling was from a combination of adrenal fatigue and impaired kidney and liver functions.]

I did go ahead with that speech, which was my first public sharing of my story. I was only on stage for ten minutes, but the response from the audience was awesome! I shared my "poop" story, which I told here in a previous chapter, and they roared with laughter. Later, quite a few people approached me to say thank you for sharing my story and that they too could relate. Maybe I am making a difference!

I have a few other speaking engagements booked for 2018. It seems a new path has emerged for me and my story. I'll be speaking to women's groups—entrepreneurs, mostly—and helping them see how life skills can be used to benefit your business. I never imagined I'd be empowering someone's business with my story of pain and illness; I only ever envisioned speaking to healthcare professionals. Is an entire new opportunity on the horizon? Maybe so. I will just have to trust God and let Him lead the way.

"In you Lord my God, I put my trust"
Psalm 25:1 (NIV)

"In all your ways submit to Him, and He will make your path straight."
Proverbs 3:6 (NIV)

Journal reflection: Are you open to opportunities that present themselves? If so, what can you do to prepare for it?

_____

_____

_____

_____

Chapter 12

Surviving loss—infertility and miscarriages

"I can do all this through him who gives me strength."
Philippians 4:13 (NIV)

I'd like to share with you our youngest son's birth story. It's a very special story that I hold dear to my heart, and one for which I praise our creator every day.

As soon as François and I married in 1996, we decided that we would try to have a baby. My husband's adorable son Mathieu was already nine by this time and was hoping for a sibling. After two years of trying, I went for exploratory surgery to see if they could find out what was wrong with me. We learned that I had a mild form of endometriosis, but nothing severe enough to prevent me from conceiving. So, the doctors put me on a fertility medication and we kept trying for another two years. Still, nothing happened. The doctors were stumped and said we should look for alternative ways to start our own family.

We tried to adopt through a Canadian organization. We went through the home study, meetings, and orientations, met all the right people, filled out all the forms, and even endured the social services evaluations and visits to our home. After this long and complicated process, the children we thought that were going to be up for adoption were now only available to foster. The government gave the birth parents the right to visitation and insisted that they would be open adoptions. There was also a chance that the child could be sent back to the birth parents, which would have been devastating for us. So, we were back to square one.

Our last hope was to try an expensive and very invasive medical procedure called in-vitro fertilisation (IVF). I had gone back to school at the University of Ottawa to become a teacher when we got the call for the IVF program. I eventually had to take a medical withdrawal from University to be able to meet the grueling schedule of appointments, procedures, and medications; my education and my degree would have to wait.

As we started IVF, we discovered that I was not the problem. François had finally been tested, and it turned out that while he had millions of "little swimmers," they were slow-moving and none of them could get to the eggs I was producing! Go figure.

My process began with multiple physical exams, followed by injections of progesterone to prepare my womb lining for the fertilised embryo. Then, I had to take other hormonal medication to trick my body into producing multiple eggs per month instead of the usual one. You women out there who complain of cramps during your monthly cycle have no idea what "cramps" really are until your ovaries are as big as softballs! The process is very complicated, but simply put I had to "force-grow" eggs. Once this phase was over, I underwent an excruciating medical procedure to retrieve the eggs. They gave me a slight sedative that pretty much wore off after fifteen minutes, and then they stuck what appeared to be a six-inch needle into my ovary. This was one of the worst experiences of my life, and I say that after having a twenty-eight-hour labour and having passed many, many kidney stones!

In the end, they managed to harvest thirteen eggs, nine of which were viable. They used a special needle under a microscope to inject François' sperm into the eggs and then into the freezer they went. Now we had to wait and see if any of them survived. The wait was agonizing.

Finally, the call came. Two of the eggs had survived! We were so excited and a little in shock, as we were possibly going to have twins!

I was to go back in five days later and have the fertilized eggs transplanted. In the meantime, I still had to take hormone medications to prepare my body for the pregnancy. Up to now the process had all been medical science—nothing natural about it. I didn't really care, though; I just wanted a baby.

However, before that could happen, I began to feel like something was not right. I was increasingly dizzy and nauseas while simultaneously feeling like I was getting weaker. François was on the RCMP Riot Troop Tactical Team at the time and was working at a demonstration for some kind of international government summit meeting in downtown Ottawa. I knew he would not be easy to get a hold of as he was at the back of the troop on the arrest team, right in the middle of the crowd. Without any family nearby, I made the unwise decision to drive myself to the hospital. I had been there often enough for fertility tests that they knew who I was and fast-tracked me through emergency and in to see the specialist. It turned out my blood pressure had dropped, and my blood work showed that my liver was reacting badly to the medication. The bad news was they wanted to postpone the transplant of the eggs as it may be too dangerous to continue. The really bad news was the eggs would not survive living out of the womb for much longer and we'd lose any chance of getting pregnant.

I was devastated, and I couldn't make this decision on my own. I needed my husband, now! I gave his pager number to the nurse and hoped François would somehow be able to contact me. While I waited, I made what I believe to be my first real prayer to God. "Please God, if you're really there, can you please let us have this baby?"

The phone call never came. Instead, this very large and panicked cop, dressed in black riot gear, showed up at the hospital demanding to see me. The doctor looked like he was going to pee himself. François had come for me! My knight in not-so-shining armour. He scared the crap out of the hospital staff, but I didn't care. The doctor decided to keep me for observation for a while and see how my lab work looked later. They finally sent me home and said everything was going to be fine, and I was cleared to undergo the final procedure. I was going to get my babies after all!

We went back to the hospital five days later, excited and nervous. The procedure to transplant the two embryos was much quicker and less painful than the retrieval. All went well, and after a brief stay I was sent home to rest. I called all of our friends and family and announced that the procedure had gone well and we would know soon if we were pregnant. Well, I say "we" were pregnant, but we all know François had the easy end of the deal!

So, we waited. And we waited. I spent some time deciding how I was going to organize the baby room. I contemplated what colors would look best with the lighting in the room and checked François' list of baby names to see if any of our favourites were the same. For a girl I wanted Geneviève, and if it was a boy François wanted Phillipe. Who knows, we might need both names!

My colour choices for the baby room kept changing. It was going to need to be something gender neutral, especially if they were going to be twins!

After supper one night, I went into the bathroom to take my medication and suddenly I experienced a horrible cramping feeling. The next thing I knew I was locking the bathroom door and blood was gushing everywhere. I made it over to the toilet, and after the bleeding stopped I looked down and screamed. I wasn't sure what I was expecting to see, but it was an image I'll never forget. I had miscarried and lost both babies.

Things were a bit of a blur after that. I only remember being depressed and feeling like I must have done something wrong. Did I move around too much after the transplant? Did I forget to take my medication? What had happened? The doctors said there was no explanation. Miscarriages are common and there is never any definitive reason. We were just unlucky. Not only had we lost our babies, but the $10,000 it cost to do the IVF procedures was non-refundable. We were now both heartbroken and broke.

You can imagine what the next few weeks were like for us, so I'll spare you the details and depressing images.

We had now spent six years trying to have a baby of our own. Don't get me wrong, I love my step-son Mathieu like he is my own. He was fifteen at the time, and we'd been raising him in our home since he was five. However, I had missed out on all the cute and cuddly baby stuff. I toyed with the idea of what would our life be like without a child of our own. Would we travel the world, buy expensive cars, and dine out at fancy restaurants? Isn't that what people with no kids do? I'd trade it all for the chance to have a little person to love, someone who would call me "Mommy."

After much thought and many, many discussions, we decided to give adoption one more try. I'd already done the research; I'm organized and almost always have a plan B.

"We're going to China!" I announced to my dumbfounded family. We had no other options left. The doctors said there was nothing else they could do to help us, and nature had already given up on us years ago. I was now thirty-two years old, and François was forty-one. The clock was ticking for both of us, and fast! It was time to make a decision.

The banks would not give us a loan for an overseas adoption, so we sucked up our pride and approached our families to see if anyone could help. Thankfully, some options were made available to us that would at least get us started. Oh happy day! It looked like our dream was finally going to become a reality. I had met some of the parents from the adoption agency and viewed many pictures of the cutest little Asian girls. Big black eyes, chubby cheeks, and jet-black hair. They were all gorgeous! I contacted the agency to find out when we had to get them the money. We also had to get all our papers in order and get some extra cash in case we had to bribe the locals; I had heard a few horror stories about getting there and running into unforeseen financial road blocks. We knew the village we were going to and wanted to name our future daughter Mia after a great female soccer player; I wanted her to have a strong namesake. Of course, we would keep her Chinese name as her middle name as we were set on making sure she knew of her Asian heritage. Suddenly, it hit me. We were really going to do this. Holy crap! We're going to China!

Around this time, I started feeling under the weather and just wasn't myself. I was working in a chiropractic office at the time and consequently was exposed to flus and colds year-round; I figured that I was probably just nauseous because I was getting sick, and that the dizziness I was feeling was most likely fatigue. One night, I was up late reading and researching books on China when the nausea got worse. It had me dry-heaving even though I hadn't been eating much.

My neighbor finally talked me into taking a pregnancy test. I thought it was a huge waste of time as the doctors had already confirmed we were not able to get pregnant, but she wouldn't stop bugging me so I bought one to shut her up. It was clearly a faulty package, because the line kept reading positive. We knew this was impossible, but she insisted I try another test. I was too sick to drive, so she went for me and came back with three more pregnancy tests. Test #2: positive. What the hell? Test #3: positive. Okay, this can be happening! Test #4: you guessed it, POSITIVE! WHAT?

It didn't make any sense. How did this happen? I mean, I knew how "it" happened, but how was I actually pregnant? I called François immediately, and he could tell something was wrong as I was sobbing into the phone. I finally calmed down and said, "I'm pregnant." The line was quiet for few seconds, and then he came back with, "Ha, that's not very funny." I passed the phone to our neighbor and she repeated what I had said. I don't really remember what he said after that; I think we were both in shock. I made an appointment and went in the next day to see a friend's doctor because mine was away. No way was I going to wait another two weeks to see if this was real or not!

At the doctor's office, I received the best news I'd ever had in my life. I was indeed pregnant! I was only three to four weeks along, so I was advised to be cautious about telling anyone in case I miscarried again. I made it a few hours before I couldn't stand it anymore and called my family with the good news.

But what about Mia? What do we do about her?

Sadly, we didn't go to China, and we would never get to meet her. We decided that going to China now that I was pregnant was a risk in itself, and my pregnancy was already at high risk, so no flying for me. It was a tough decision, because if I had a miscarriage we couldn't go back and change our minds. However, I couldn't think like that; I was too happy about the fact that I was miraculously pregnant with our own baby! Praise God!

Years later, I would have some feelings of regret about not going to get Mia. I felt like we had abandoned her. I had lost yet another child that I already loved but would never get to hold. I remember all the photos of Chinese infants, and I could visualize her face with her chubby little cheeks and shining black hair. She would have been eighteen months old at the time we signed adoption papers. Today, she would be about seventeen. I thought that she would be like me, playing sports, ignoring boys, and goofing around with friends. Her favourite sport would be softball, same as mine.

I remember feeling sad that we never got to meet her. I would pray for her and hope that whoever did adopt her loved and cherished her. I still think of her from time to time and feel a slight tug of regret. However, I know in my heart that God has made sure she was taken care of somehow, and I take peace and comfort in this knowledge.

"The Lord is close to the brokenhearted and saves those who are crushed in spirit."
Psalm 34:18 (NIV)

The nine months that I carried our son Ben were very stressful as I was afraid of losing yet another baby. My days were full of morning sickness, although really it was more like all-day sickness. François brought me soda crackers to my bedside each morning and I would have to sit still for a bit, try a few crackers, and then get out of bed. My doctor put me on an anti-nausea medication made specifically for pregnancies. I was so ill that I only gained eighteen pounds for the entire pregnancy, which I have to admit I was a little grateful about. However, the aftermath of twenty-eight hours of labour and a fourth-degree tear that required two repair surgeries wasn't something I was expecting. I guess it was a small price to pay for our miracle baby.

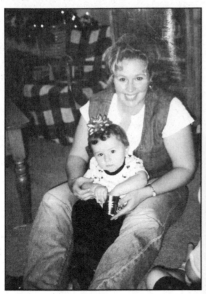

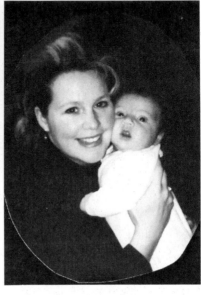

Post-partum depression (PPD) kicked in a few short weeks later, and at the time I didn't recognize how dangerous it could be. I remember leaving Ben on the living room floor when he was only a few months old, walking out of the house to the neighbor's place, and telling her to go take care of him because I was afraid I would hurt him somehow. I didn't have any family out east and my husband's family were two and a half hours away in Montreal. I had no one to turn to except for my dear friend Nancy, whom I am forever grateful to for taking care of both of me and our baby. She had three kids and was a pro at calming me and the baby down.

I started sneaking a glass of wine at 10 a.m., trying to steady my nerves. Little did I know that I would meet many mothers who would share similar stories and tell me what their go-to vices were!

The difficult part for me was the guilt. I had waited seven years for this baby, and now that he was here, I didn't always want to be around him. I finally had to admit to my doctor that I was having terrifying and strange visions of injuring him. We needed to fix this, and fast!

Many women suffer with "baby blues" and emotional periods of sadness, fatigue, and self-doubt after having a baby. This condition usually subsides in two to three weeks' time. However, if these symptoms last longer than that, it could be a more serious condition such as PPD. This can be extremely harmful for both mother and baby if it isn't treated promptly and correctly by medical professionals. I finally gave in and went for counselling, but I was resentful about having to go. After all, I was trained in Critical Incident Stress Management and other Disaster Response techniques. I could jump on a plane with a backpack and end up in another country helping with hurricane relief. How can I not deal with this little baby?

It was mindboggling to me and so incredibly frustrating to both myself and François.

It didn't help that I couldn't sleep because I needed to hear him breathing. When I did finally get to sleep, he would wake up crying. The sleep deprivation alone was debilitating. If you're a parent, you know what I'm talking about.

I did recover after a while and have a lot of wonderful memories with Ben in the first year, but I'll admit that it was struggle. I went back to work when Ben was six months old; I wasn't meant to be a stay-at-home mom, not yet anyway. Thankfully, François was able to take paternity leave and cover off the other six months at home with the baby.

Mathieu, our older son, was fifteen at the time and would be learning to drive in a few short months. Picture having one child driving a car, while at the same time your other child isn't even walking yet! Having a teenager and a baby at the same time was quite the adventure. Mathieu was such a great big brother, though, and was very helpful in taking care of his baby brother.

The pair of them now both stand six feet tall. Ben is fifteen and Mathieu is thirty, and although they are separated in distance, their hearts are always connected in brotherly love. It's fun to see them now at different stages of their lives. We are so incredibly proud of both our boys; they've become amazing people with kind hearts and sharp minds, each of them with their own unique talents and gifts.

Ben wrote me this lovely and enlightening sonnet this year for his English class. Ben included his interpretation in brackets, insightful for a fifteen-year-old. He stole my title, the brat!

"Comfortable Pain"
by Benjamin Cadotte, Grade 10, (age 15)

What is comfortable pain,
It's waking up every morning feeling agony.
       (feeling pain)
Or is it the chill down your spine in the rain,
       (rain can cause arthritis to be more severe)
Pain is cost/worth more than money.
       (cost a lot money to manage pain)
So might I touch with a single finger,
       (the slight touch of a finger)
It shall feel as harmful as a giant needle:
       (feels super painful)
A single crackle of thunder could even trigger,
       (jolting up when getting scared, hurts)
The pain inside that isn't so gleeful.
Modernized sweets are the only solution to my dilemma,
       (drugs/medication)
Although a flaw causes me to grow.
       (causes weight gain)
Sometimes I feel as pretty as Princess Leia,
       (feeling happy because of the really strong medication)
Sometimes my head spins in an uneasy flow.
       (you get lots of headaches and head spins)
Have no fear the man is near,
       (don't be scared, God is near)
To make sure you hear through the right ear.
       (to help guide you)

Wow, what can I say? I cried, I laughed, I hugged my boy! What an amazing heart he has. I felt some guilt knowing what all my health issues have cost him, but I think I felt love the most; my heart just overflowed when I first read this. Maybe he's become such a compassionate soul because of my illnesses? I'd like to think so. It proves to me that God's grace all around us.

Journal reflection: Are you holding onto any regrets, or are you able to forgive yourself and let go?

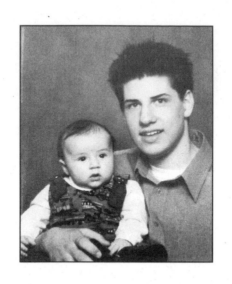

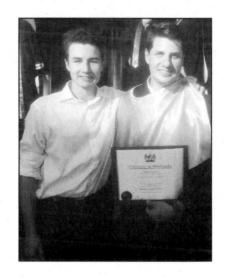

Chapter 13

Caregiving and self-care

Being a caregiver is one of the most rewarding things you can ever do for someone. I think that's what connected with me the most about being a nurse; I considered it a privilege to care for someone who was in pain, or who had just come out of the operating room and was recovering from surgery, or even someone who was facing a terminal illness. What a blessing, to be there for their last breath. The rewards are priceless; however, a lack of self-care can lead to "caregiver burnout."

Even medically-trained professionals that have received extensive education and training can struggle to work under this kind of day-to-day trauma and total care for someone in hospital. Now, imagine having to care for someone you know and love in a home setting; it can be a daunting situation. I'm sure if you ask François, he would say he had no idea the beginning of his retirement would involve being a caregiver to his wife, the nurse.

"Carry each other's burdens, and in this way you will fulfill the law of Christ."
Galatians 6:2 (NIV)

Maintaining independence is something most of us take for granted, right up until you have to rely on someone else to do something for you. When I first went on medical leave in 2015, I had already been struggling to walk or sit for long periods of time. I was looking into traction and other torturous treatments to help improve my physical symptoms, but being at home full time was one of the most difficult changes to overcome. At the time, we didn't know this would be the end of my nursing career. We had hoped it was just a break from my stressful work environment. I loved my job, and I was really good at it; my body, however, had other plans. It was tired. The lupus, fibromyalgia, osteoarthritis, and a host of other flare-ups were relentless, and they were taking me down hard and fast.

Our home life became stressful as we were still raising a busy teenager, and throwing a chronically ill person into the mix made things a bit complicated. François was a trooper though! He stepped up like nobody's business and took over almost everything in terms of maintaining the household, including cooking, laundry, groceries, dog walking, vacuuming, and anything else that needed taking care of. If it needed to be done, he did it, no questions asked.

François is my primary caregiver. There are times when my pain is excruciating and mobility is limited, and he has to help me get dressed. He'll complain, "This is so stupid, I should be taking your bra off, not putting it back on!" Often, a string of very bad French words follows.

For almost two years, driving was something of a rare occasion for me. The disc degeneration in my neck prevented me from being able to perform a shoulder check or get my seat belt on. I would lose strength in my arms, or my hands wouldn't work, or I couldn't get my hip to lift into the car. During this time, François had to be the one who get everyone where we needed to go.

Other times, the family decision making—something we have always done as a team—would be placed completely on François shoulders. Thank goodness he has a pretty big set of shoulders!

I often would tell François to get out of the house and spend some time with his other love—his Vintage Indian motor bike. He works hard at home and makes sure everyone gets what they need, so he deserves some time to himself. My job is to make sure he gets a break from being the caregiver to his wife and has some time to do something he enjoys.

I know how lucky I am to have him. We've been together twenty-seven years now, and this blow really could have damaged our marriage. Not only were we dealing with my illness and disability, we were facing a significant loss of income. My paycheck only continued until the end of my sick leave, and then there was nothing. I've heard of other marriages breaking up over less, which is so incredibly sad.

Our marriage has made it through this trial. We are together in sickness and health, just like the vows we took on our wedding day. I'm so proud of François for setting an example to our boys. This is how a reliable and caring husband shows love and commitment to his wife and his marriage, no matter what! How blessed I am!

June 24, 2016

I went shopping today at Laura and spent three hours trying on clothes. Most of the clothes came from the plus size area, and I wasn't thrilled to be on that side of the store. However, it is what it is, and having new clothes and feeling beautiful was the goal. In the end I was happy with the choices, François got to see them all, and my visa got a good work out! I couldn't believe how much I enjoyed having these new clothes—I couldn't stop smiling! This may sound shallow to some people, but when you're in pain or sick all the time, looking good is not a priority. Your self-confidence takes a hit when the only thing that you can manage to put on is a t-shirt and yoga pants. Self-care takes a bit of back seat when you're ill, because your focus is on managing the pain. As trivial as it may sound to some, even brushing your teeth and a washing your face before bed can become a daunting workout.

Tonight was a treat though! I got to hang out with our good friend and neighbor Lorraine and my hubby François at the pub. An outing like this is rare for me these days. However, it is "Ste. Jean Baptise", a special Quebec holiday, so we must celebrate, especially as François and Lorraine are both French-Canadian! Shopping, a night out with people that make me laugh…today was a great day! I'm grateful for pretty clothes that fit well and for some much-needed laughter. A day for celebration indeed!

I am beautiful, and I am loved.

～

Whether you are a caregiver or the person being cared for, it is extremely important to practice self care. As a caregiver, this is the best way to reduce the risk of burnout and make sure that you can continue caring for your loved one. As the person being cared for, this ensures that you stay in the best health possible and helps reduce how much care you need.

I always figured I was two steps ahead of the average person when it came to healing oneself, because I was a nurse who was also living with chronic pain and multiple autoimmune diseases. What I wasn't willing to hear or be open to, however, was that I myself had been causing a lot of the issues. Sure, I was healthy for years, an outstanding athlete, and educated in health and nutrition, but did I practice what I was preaching? The simple answer was no, I did not. Not as well as I could be. It was so much easier to blame the diseases, the medications, my genetics, my personal problems, and so on. But, even though I had good medical practitioners and a contact list full of reputable specialists who were top in their field, I just kept getting sicker. I realized had been lying to myself, and I was not taking care of this body God had given me to protect and honour. I had some serious questions to ask myself:

- Was I being accountable for how I treated my body?
- Did I make an effort to make sure I put in only good food and nutrition?
- Did I rest when I needed to?
- Did I stop working or slow down when I should have?
- Did I value my titles, my status, and my position more than my health?
- Did I believe the medication was the only way to manage all the diseases I had acquired?
- Did I accept my illnesses and give up on myself?

These are questions I would like you to consider about yourself. Going through these will give you a better idea of whether you are truly doing everything you can to take care of yourself, or if you're just making excuses. Below, I've included some of the approaches I've found the most useful in taking care of my physical and mental health.

How I changed it all

To reduce fatigue, I started taking naps during the day, usually between 3:00-4:00 p.m. for anywhere between thirty to sixty minutes. I don't do this every day, but if my body needs it I will.

Improving my nutrition was also a big step. Unfortunately for me, I'm a stress eater. That means if I get stressed, I eat, even if I'm not hungry. Obviously, weight gain is an ongoing issue. I have, however, been able to address the issue and plan better for times when I am overly stressed. I have connections to some amazing people that work in nutrition, and they have given me some great tips. One of the best things is to stay hydrated! You must drink lots of water, every hour if you can. Water has many benefits, including filling you up, and it also gives your skin a nice healthy glow. Another good approach is to keep healthy snacks prepared and ready to eat.

I started paying attention to vitality coach Barb Wallick. She is a licenced Food and Spirit practitioner, among a multitude of other things, whom practices what she preaches. I've witnessed her transformation into a healthy, balanced, well-rounded individual. She counselled me on some of the foods that may cause inflammation (mainly sugar) and helped me learn to identify healthier alternatives.

I also have to give a shout out to Brenda Eastwood, RNCP, for her guidance with the right vitamin and mineral supplements. Ask Brenda and she'll confess I was one of the most difficult cases she's ever worked with. Understanding all my unique symptoms and the supplements I had to avoid was quite a challenge. She advised me on the proper vitamins such as B, C, D, and once we had that out then there were the hormones and pain levels to deal with. Magnesium was a big help with pain and sleep. Leveling out my cortisol levels really helped with moods swings and weight gain. Just a reminder here to always check with your doctor to make sure these supplements won't interfere with any prescription medication you may be taking.

Taking part in something you enjoy is also extremely beneficial. At one point, I found myself skipping out on a yoga class or missing out on movie night, two things I love but don't always feel confident in attending. There have been so many times I've really wanted to just stay home because it was less stressful and less work than getting there. I have learned to go anyway, have some fun, and hang out with some people so we could spend time together. It's important to keep some guilt-free fun in your life; you deserve it!

For me, music has always been one of my best healing tools. One song that helped me get through a particular rough patch was called "Just be held", by Casting Crowns. The lyrics include, "You're not alone, stop holding on and just be held. Your world's not falling apart, it's falling into to place." These words give me comfort, reassuring me that God is in control and that I need to trust that and stop trying to do it all on my own. I also get goose bumps when people sing. It's all so healing and touches my heart, reminding me of when I used to sing in a band and of the women's ministry choir at my church.

When I want to practice calm and peacefulness, I retreat to my back yard in the warmer months. Thank goodness for the Creator's splendour of nature. I find so much peace in my garden and my back deck, and I enjoy making them beautiful with flowers, herbs, rocks, driftwood, and seashells that I have collected from numerous beaches. The hot tub and the hammock are a welcome site, but my favourite spot is the wooden Adirondack chair beside my water fountain. I have my coffee there every morning, so long as the sun is out, from April to September. The birds call to each other, although I sometimes I think they are talking to me. In the evening we light the fire—okay, it's propane, but it's still a wonderful way to sit with friends and have a glass of wine. In the cooler, rainier months, I'm fireside in my living room on our soft leather couch, accompanied by my favorite blanket, our dog Cooper, and my essential oil diffuser.

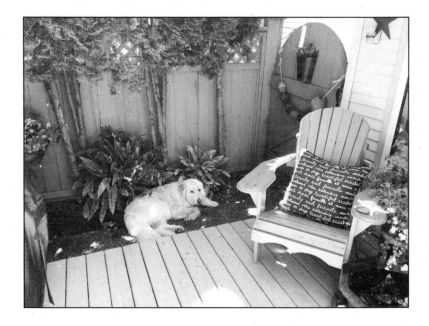

Everyone needs to be pampered once in a while. I'm extremely grateful to the hairstylists who have been doing my hair since my lupus diagnosis in 2005. I love coming to see them and being pampered; a nice hair cut is good for your self-esteem, and looking good is always a bonus when you feel like crap.

Sometimes, what I find most helpful is writing in my journal or enjoying a good book or movie. François and I love movies; they just have a way of transporting you to another time and place, allowing me to keep my spirit feeling full and happy. Giving ourselves time to relax and have fun is critical to our mental health!

Another approach that has had a huge impact is practicing the "Law of Attraction." This concept comes from a book of the same name, written by Michael J. Losier, and is about "the science of attracting more of what you want and less of what you don't want." For example, instead of saying "I don't want to be *sick*," say "I want to be *healthy*." Your unconscious mind and the vibrations of the universe only hear the key word of what it is that you want. So, if it only hears you asking for "sick," you get more of being sick. Change your focus to "healthy" and that's what you'll get more of. Say "I want to have lots of *energy*" instead of "I don't want to be *tired* anymore." Say "I am getting *stronger*" instead of "I'm so *weak*." Following this practice has really helped me stay in a positive state of mind. Try it; you'll be pleasantly surprised by the results!

Make a check list!

My husband calls me "the list lady," and that's probably an accurate description. With memory loss as one of the many side effects of multiple chronic illness, pain, and medications, lists have become my friend. I chose to accept my memory loss and make myself accountable for what I need to do keep my own self-care in check, so I created the following list:

1. **Pain control:** stay on top of your pain levels so they don't get away from you. Don't tough it out as this prolongs healing.
2. **Medication:** make sure you take your medications correctly and on time. They don't work as well if they're not taken when prescribed
3. **Nutrition:** this is a major line of defense in fighting illness. Prep healthy meals and snacks ahead of time so they're easy to access on difficult days
4. **Meditation/ Prayer:** our spiritual health is what keeps us grounded. Deep breathing counts!
5. **Exercise:** participating in activities such as restorative yoga (my favourite), swimming, or even a short walk also keeps your mental health in check.
6. **Rest:** pace yourself, especially if you have an event, work, or errands to run later in the day.
7. **Treatment:** look into physiotherapy, chiropractors, registered massage therapy (not the spa kind), acupuncture, or whatever else helps you manage your symptoms.
8. **Counselling/coaching:** this provides you with a professional and objective listener who can offer you new coping skills .

~

July 14, 2016

Meditation is something new I'm trying. Emphasis, however, is on the word "trying." I can't help but roll my eyes every time I start out. I either can't get my current pain under control to focus on relaxing, or I can't quiet down the persistent ridiculous thoughts I have in my head that won't stop spinning out of control; sometimes, it's both at once.

There are thousands of meditation CDs and apps out there. I tried a few that were recommended to me, but I usually turn them off after the first ninety seconds because I can't stand the annoyingly monotone voice of the narrator.

Recently I was introduced to Deepak Chopra and his Quantum healing, and if I can follow his instructions it might just work with reducing my pain levels. There are books and CD's available, but I found some great videos on YouTube for free. Who doesn't like free? If nothing else, it has helped with my anxiety.

Upon passing a very large kidney stone yesterday, I contemplated whether or not the stone was "released pain and disbeliefs" that my body and mind allowed me to let go of after finishing a Neuro-Linguistic Programming Timeline coaching session with my friend, Teri Holland. I feel so much better physically and emotionally than I have in a long while. Although I did experience a gastritis attack this evening, I'm happier than I have been in months. I feel like a strong sense of peace has been blanketed over me. I have so much hope that I will be healed of all my illnesses and pain.

I haven't got all the answers for how to take care of yourself and your chronic illness, but what I do know is that having a chronic illness or living in constant pain—or any other life struggle, for that matter—is no picnic. Know what your limitations are and how much can you take before you hit a breaking point. If you aren't familiar with what your signals to slow down are, maybe you're not listening to your own inner voice or paying attention to what your body is trying to tell you. Maybe it's not a voice; maybe it's a feeling or an emotion that persists no matter how much you try to distract yourself from it.

Be kind to yourself. Be aware of your mind, body, and spirit. Does one of them need nurturing? Do you need to rest? Do you need a break from whatever is causing the stress? Most likely, you can see or feel when you've run out of steam. However, for those of us living with chronic illnesses, knowing when to put the brakes on can be difficult and unclear. I caution you to heed the warning signs. If your stubbornness to "not give in" is making you sicker or causing you more pain, then it's time to revaluate which battles you want to be fighting. It's important to pace yourself; what you do today will dictate what you are able to do tomorrow.

For both caregivers and people being cared for, it is imperative that you make sure you have access to the resources you need to meet your current needs. This could mean assistive devices for your loved one or having emotional support for yourself. It's always best to have a least one person you can share your feelings with. You or your family member might require professional help if feelings become too dark or depression is suspected. Don't be afraid to reach out and ask for help.

We've all heard the emergency announcement they use on the airplane "in case of emergency and the air bags drop down, please put your own oxygen mask on first, then you may assist those around you." This applies to our everyday life as well. You are of no use to anyone if you can't take care of yourself! One of my favorite mantras is, "You can be replaced at work, but not at home." I'm not exactly sure where I heard this, but it's so true for all of us. Have you ever seen a tombstone with the engravings of someone's job title? "Here lies the responsible CEO?" Doesn't it usually read, "Here lays our loving wife/husband and mother/father?" Making what matters most a priority is so essential to our well-being.

Caring for someone can be a wonderful experience, but it can also cause and enormous amount of stress on you and your relationships. We need to allow ourselves some downtime to prevent burnout; this is absolutely necessary in order to be able to continue providing care. The symptoms of burnout are similar to the signs of depression and can come in a wide variety and range; from minor to severe, and from physical to emotional. Here are some of the signs and symptoms to watch for if you are a caregiver:

- Changes in sleep patterns (sleeping too much or not enough)
- Changes in appetite, weight, or both (either overeating and weight gain or undereating and weight loss)
- No interest in things you used to love to do
- Not participating in activities or going out
- Having a sense of hopelessness
- Feeling like you have no control over your situation
- Feelings of guilt for taking time for yourself

If you recognize the signs and symptoms of depression or anxiety/panic attacks, you have some options in terms of seeking help. If you are imminent danger, such as experiencing strong suicidal thoughts, call your local emergency line for immediate help. The Canadian Association for Suicide Prevention (www.suicideprevention.ca) and Life Line Foundation Canada (www.thelifelinecanada.ca) can also connect you with crisis centers in your area. If you are not in crisis but are at risk of burning out, there are educational courses, counselling, and supports group that are available to you and can help you better take care of yourself. In Canada, your local public health department can provide you with the options closest to you.

> **Journal reflection:** How do you reach out for support when you're feeling overwhelmed? How do you show kindness to yourself?
>
> _____
>
> _____
>
> _____
>
> _____

Chapter 14

Gratitude is the attitude

Being able to express gratitude is such a gift. There is a quote by William Arthur Ward that goes, "Feeling gratitude and not expressing it is like wrapping a gift and not giving it." This is one of the main reasons I started writing a journal; it helps me reflect on the important things in my life. Noticing and appreciating the things I do have instead of the things that I don't is easier when I write them down and express thankfulness for those gifts.

Having a positive attitude can be so challenging when you live with chronic illnesses and debilitating pain. In order to survive, it's imperative that we learn to practice maintaining a positive outlook. There are some questions that we need to ask ourselves: do I really need more than what I already have? How can I let people l know I appreciate them more? One place to start is being kind to ourselves and to others. There's also a saying that goes, "Kindness is a language which the deaf can hear and the blind can see." I love this quote! To me, it means that if you give of your heart, material things that you can see or touch don't matter.

Starting a gratitude journal

A gratitude journal can be typed or handwritten. I find the latter to be more creative because you can add drawings and make it an "artistic journal." I bought myself a ring-bound paper journal and some fun colour markers to write in and add colours or sketch designs. Here are some tips for keeping a gratitude journal:

- **Routine:** they say it takes twenty-one days to form a habit, so find a routine and stick with it, such as writing every night before bedtime. It gets easier by day fourteen.
- **Make it personal:** write things for your eyes only; self-disclosure helps reduce stress.
- **Gifts:** be grateful for gifts you have (family, friends, love, faith) rather than dwelling on the things you don't have

On the next page are some entries from my journal that demonstrate how I practice gratitude, as well as a letter to myself which was a practice exercise I did to acknowledge my gratitude for all that I already have.

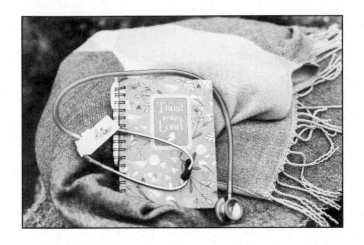

~

June 21, 2016

Pain levels were very high today, 8/10. However, I had a real emotional breakthrough. I was able to release some past anger, sadness, fear, and hurt. Hurt was the hardest one to let go of—I cried while fighting with it. I was so exhausted afterward. I was supposed to have a bible study night with my sister, but I was left too emotionally exhausted to do both in the same day. My gratitude for today: letting go of past emotions, my sister's compassion, and my RMT treatment which, although painful, was very helpful.

~

June 16, 2016

Had a great session of self-discovery today with my Neurolinguistics Language Practitioner and Timeline coach,

Teri Holland. We went through a process to discover my main values. I came up with three values: Thrive, Empower, and Love.

Our plan is as follows. First, I will continue to journal daily. Second, I will add three things I'm grateful for. Third, I will write positive affirmations starting with "I am..." Fourth, I will make a vision board with my three new discovered values.

Another method I learned from Teri is the ancient Hawaiian practice of forgiveness called "Ho'oponopono." Traditionally it was a practice used by Indigenous Hawaii healers, and today there's a new practice that goes by the same name. There are four steps to this process that you do on your own, whenever you want. No need for anyone to hear you, except you. You can say it to yourself or you could write it in your journal.

Step 1: Repentance. "I'm sorry."

Step 2: Ask forgiveness. "Please forgive me."

Step 3: Gratitude. "Thank you."

Step 4: Love. "I love you!"

When we forgive others for past hurts or disappointments, it doesn't have to be face-to-face. Some of our friends and family may not be at peace the issue at hand, and part of the healing process is for you to forgive them, even if they don't know they have been forgiven. Then you can move forward and not let the past block you from moving forward.

Love is very present in my home today. My wonderful husband and I discussed how stress is one of my major contributors to illness.

My gratitude today is for François and his love for me, for the sun and its warmth, and for my super fluffy Goldendoodle Cooper, who stayed beside me all day today with unconditional love.

～

June 30, 2016
Letter to myself: Changing My Story—My Ideal day

I wake up to the sound of birds singing. My Goldendoodle Cooper stretches and takes up the entire end of the bed, but he looks so comfortable that I don't dare move this furry bundle of cuteness. I turn my head and see my wonderful husband beside me. **I praise God** for allowing him to be in my life. François is the centre of my universe, my rock, and my true love.

I pray with gratitude for the sun peeking in through my widow, the breath that I am breathing, the thoughts that I am thinking, and for all the beautifulness God has given us to live in.

I breathe deeply and imagine my body healing itself as the cells regenerate and build healthy tissue, overcoming all illness, all disease, and all pain. **I see myself as strong and determined**, ready to face the day. **I breathe deeply**, get dressed, and feel beautiful. My heart rises above any negative energy, protects me from going down the dark path of my illness, and leads me to my **new path of healing, wellness, and happiness with myself**, just as I am. Knowing I am doing the best I can with what I have, and that I will continue to **thrive and not just survive** . I drink a glass of water.

I am grateful for my thirteen-year-old son Benjamin and his wonderful laughter; it reminds me of our older son Mathieu and how his laughter was the same laugh at that age. I remind myself of the good memories of the past days we have had as a family, and I promise **to create more wonderful memories**. They hold my heart and mean more to me than anything else in the world. **How lucky I am** that my boys are healthy, smart, funny, kind, and compassionate young men. I'm so proud to be their mom.

I command my soul to feel love, to give love, and to show love to each person I encounter today. **I give thanks** for the amazing women that have supported me, and for the family and friends that continue to have faith in my ability to rise above.

I am proud of myself for enduring the physical and emotional pain. **I thank God again** for bringing me through these difficult times, and then I smile knowing He already knew I was going to be okay.

I drink a healthy protein shake and feel the minerals and proteins providing my body with sustenance. My daily medication is waiting for me. As I look at them, I know they are necessary for now, but envision how wonderful it will be to not have to take them anymore. **My body will heal itself** and won't need the medication. **I breathe** and prepare to drive to physio. I do not use my cane but put it into the trunk of my car just in case. As I park in the handicapped spot, **I remind myself this is only temporary**. I will not be parking here forever. It does **not matter what other people think**. They do not know my story, but they will soon. I feel the necessary pain of the traction machine, but praise God that I have been given the opportunity to have trained professionals that help me to heal properly. I do the therapy and **imagine my body to be pain free**. As I pay for my appointment, I am grateful for my husband's insurance, for without it, our lives would be extremely difficult.

I return home to look at my garden and sit in **my sacred space**: my Adirondack chair beside my little fish pond. I listen to the water fountain bubbling softly and allow the tension in my back to release. I close my eyes and **listen again to nature, thanking God** for creating such and amazing environment for us to live in. Cooper sits beside me, giving his affection and hoping it to be returned, and it is. His presence is so therapeutic, **so loving and calming**. I drink more water. The fish look up at me for food; I happily provide it to them. I am entranced as they swim in circles in the water and dive deep to retrieve the food I have given them.

As I check my emails, I remind myself to be okay with whatever messages I receive. **I will be okay when I am asked to prove my symptoms, and I will not see the words as accusations or judgement.** I am not in control of the world; **I do not have all the answers**, nor shall I try to do so. I will just be me as I am now. I drink more water.

Dinner will be a joint effort between my husband and I. We choose protein and salad with yet another a tall glass of ice water, the sixth or seventh of the day. **We pray together and give thanks** to the Lord for providing us with nourishment for our bodies and for **protecting us through our day**. We **ask God for healing** and say "Amen". We eat and recall moments of the day.

After dinner, **I choose to ignore my fatigue** and we take Cooper for a walk to the park. I get tired and we sit on a park bench. We smile as we watch others play or greet us with their dogs.

I am grateful to be home and ready to put my swollen feet up for a **well-deserved break** and enjoy my lemon water. I am, however, proud for going out for a walk and getting the exercise; even if it was for a short amount of time, **I still did it**. I will **take it as a win** and a moment of moving forward to a better and healthier me.

I will write small amounts in my journal, knowing that **these entries will be part of my future**. The book I am writing will include these writings and change my story from **being a debilitated patient into being the healthy, vibrant,** and amazing women that I know I am capable of. The world needs me to be an example of what courage and determination can do. I will get healthy and move towards **the happier and more energizing lifestyle** that I deserve.

I see myself on stage in front of a crowd of women. We are laughing together, and I'm having fun. When I'm finished, **I have many women come over to meet me** and we enjoy our time together. I will be blessed by the ability to inspire others and learn from them and their stories. **We build a connection.** We form a bond of powerful and **amazing friendships and opportunities**.

I can't wait for this to become a reality. For today I will drink my water and **tell the universe what I need**. I will ask God for healing and see myself as once again being a **strong, happy, healthy, and successful** person who inspires others to achieve their potential.

I wash my face and use a light **lavender mist for calming**. I love how my skin feels clean and fresh and has made it through another wonderful day. As **I pray and give thanks for my day**, Cooper hops up onto the bed and snuggles in with us for the night. We won't have a lot of room, but we don't care. We just feel loved.

~

There are so many creative ways to experience gratitude. I've mentioned a vision board, the gratitude journal, ancient tribal practices, and prayer as ways to express ourselves. If you can take time every day to appreciate what you already have instead of what you don't, you're on your way to overcoming the negative vibe that living with chronic illness and pain have.

I believe we can thrive with illness, as much of an oxymoron as that sounds. We have our bad days and we have our good days, but we'd never see the good days if not for the bad ones. What I do know is this; we have the capacity to find balance and allow ourselves forgiveness on the days that we need more care. It is however, up to us to declare that we need extra care some days and give ourselves permission to receive that care wholeheartedly, without feelings of guilt.

"Praise be to the Lord, to God our Saviour, who daily bears our burden."
Psalm 68:19 (NIV)

Journal reflection: How do you show gratitude to friends and family?

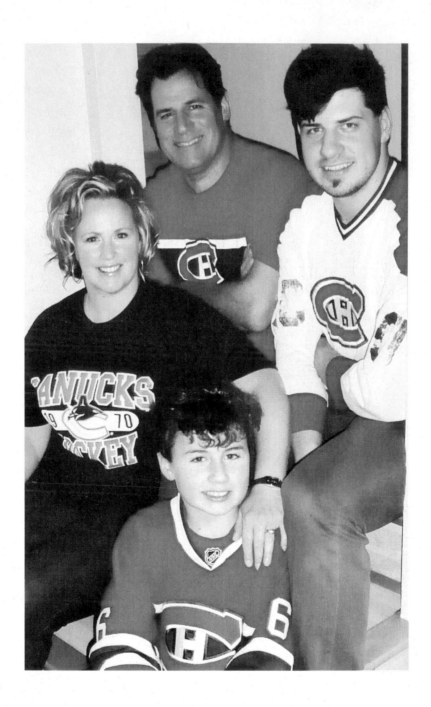

Chapter 15

Ridiculous remedies

Have you ever had someone give you unsolicited advice when you're sick or injured? I get it, people want to help in their own way. It makes sense for them to think they're helping by sharing grandma's secret recipe for treating a flu or cold. That being said, how is it that someone who has no personal experience with debilitating pain and severe fatigue thinks they could possibly understand what it's like? I don't really know, but there seems to be a lot of advice from these kinds of people anyway.

Our friends and family love us and want to help, but they may have no understanding of what we are going through. Remember to be kind when they share their "remedies," as they may have no other way of telling you they care. You could, however, let them know what your boundaries are, such as saying that unsolicited advice is not welcome nor open for discussion.

The burden usually falls on us to explain what we can about our condition in simple terms. If this is a new diagnosis for you, let people know that you're still learning and don't have all the answers. Refer those close to you to a credible website if you don't feel you can comfortably explain your situation to them. Or, better yet, sit down and look at the information together. I'm a nurse and an educator, so I've been quite comfortable with teaching my friends and family, but it's good for them to know there is more information out there. There is always the possibility that someone or some site describes it better. I always like to use something that gives a visual; as they say, a picture is worth a thousand words. Beware of Dr. Google, though; there's plenty of garbage on the internet that's inaccurate and not up to date. I've included some resources at the back of this book that you may find helpful.

Even something as simple as feeling pain can become complicated when you have a chronic illness. Our individual perception of pain is so incredibly different from person to person. The emotions and experiences as to why we feel pain are difficult to understand, and dealing with multiple sources of pain makes the situation even more complicated. Half the time I don't even realize something hurts until the other major hurt goes away. Then I'm left going "oh crap, why is this bothering me now," when in fact that pain has been there all along. There are times when I'm honestly not sure what the cause of the pain is; it's hard to pinpoint the source when competing illnesses and symptoms are so similar.

My "favourite" is when someone that knows me well sees me limping or looking uncomfortable and asks me, "What did you do?" I think to myself, do I be polite and kindly remind them that I've lived with lupus for over thirteen years while quietly cursing under my breath? No, nope, can't call them an idiot, that would be counterproductive and not helpful to the cause. Just call them "idiots" in your head and try not to let it show on your face. It's not their fault that they keep forgetting every week that I've had lupus for *thirteen years* and that's why I feel shitty. They couldn't know that you can simply wake up with symptoms without having done anything. That it's your immune system attacking you. You can sleep twelve hours and get up feeling like you just ran a marathon. You're so beat up, it's almost not fair that you didn't even get to have any fun doing something you shouldn't have the night before!

Below are some of the unsolicited recommendations and comments I've been given to help me "get over" my chronic illnesses.

"Try to be a more positive person." If you really know me and what I've been through, you'll realize that I probably couldn't be any more of a positive person than I already am.

"You can't be that sick, you look fine." Disability doesn't always mean a wheelchair, and most chronic illnesses are invisible. Just because I look fine doesn't mean I feel fine; I put a lot of effort into appearing "normal" when I'm out in public.

"You should exercise every day. No pain, no gain!" Wrong! Pain is not gain, especially when you are chronically ill. It's our body telling us to stop. Yes, exercise is important, but remember that there is no one-size-fits-all with chronic illness. Individual activity levels need to be carefully assessed and assigned accordingly by your GP, Rheumatologist, Physiotherapist, or other specialists. You may need more rest during flare ups as overexertion can exacerbate them, leaving you worse off than before you exercised or pushed an activity beyond what you intended. Ignore what other people are saying or doing; we don't play by the same set of rules. We have to protect ourselves from trying to please others just to appear "normal." This *is* our normal! Own it and protect it, or you'll pay for it.

Getting outside, breathing fresh air, and being in nature is healing. Slow and steady wins every time. Just get out there, even if it's only for a ten-minute walk, because it gets you dressed and out of the house! Swimming is also fantastic for your joints and mobility. For many of us, it's a struggle to find the courage to put on a bathing suit and go out in public. Just do it! Sorry, but you're not so special that they will have a red carpet and paparazzi hanging out poolside, waiting for you to reveal your bathing suit. Not going to happen.

Recently I've started doing Restorative Yoga, where you hold yourself in positions with the support of bolsters and blankets. You stretch at your own pace and ability, and it's so relaxing. If you get a good instructor, they will transition the poses slowly so you don't feel like you're falling behind. This is a sacred space for you to unwind, clear your head, and just breathe and be grateful to your body for getting you there. Namaste.

"Just eat raw green leafy vegetables, they're good for everything." They can also be one of the main culprits for causing kidney stones, which for me are usually followed by an infection and have caused me to be hospitalized more than I care to mention. I've been fighting with kidney stones for over twenty years, so I think I qualify as experienced on the subject.

"You should take Echinacea, it's a natural immune booster." Sure is, and is completely contraindicated by my lupus medication, which is taken to supress my already hyperactive immune system.

"You should try going off all prescription drugs, that should help balance out your system." I'm sorry, where did you say you got your got your medical degree? Don't listen to people to that have no experience—it can be so dangerous. DO NOT GO COLD TURKEY OFF YOUR MEDS! I've seen other people try this many years ago and it was not pretty; they got very sick!

Lupus and fibromyalgia are extremely complicated and incurable diseases. They haven't received a lot of publicity, and therefore not enough awareness or funding for research is available. It was only a few short years ago that most doctors actually started recognizing that fibromyalgia is not an imaginary condition made up by hypochondriacs. We're just scratching the surface here, folks; there so much more we need to learn about these types of conditions.

I can remember the first time I mentioned my fibromyalgia symptoms to a former doctor, who laughed at me and said it was all in my head. Another brilliant doctor said he had no time for non-existent, imaginary illnesses, and that I was wasting his time. It was one of the most traumatizing times in my life, almost worse than the pain and fatigue itself. How horrible for someone to think that you had nothing better to do but make up fake symptoms. It's so ridiculous and upsetting. Please don't give up! Your body is worth fighting for!

Don't be afraid to educate your doctor. They are just humans, not God. They may not have come across your combination of symptoms before and may need to look into your clinical symptoms before they decide what needs to be done. Or, you may need to see a specialist. A lot of what is involved with making a diagnosis is process of elimination, so it's important that they ask you lots of questions. Don't forget to make notes at home and have them ready for your appointment. If you haven't found the right health care team, keep looking!

Thank goodness there are many caring physicians that listen to their patients and haven't forgotten the compassion they learned in medical school. I've been incredibly lucky to have finally found an amazing Rheumatologist and GP that take me seriously and listen to what I have to say. They've seen how far I have come and how quickly it can go south.

It really is a team effort.

I caution you not to go it alone; make sure you save yourself and your family some grief by finding some professional support. My doctors and I make a point of setting some realistic goals for me to achieve in a timely manner that aren't too stressful. My goals can be related to nutrition, exercise, new medication dosages, rest, daily activity, or the introduction of physiotherapy treatment. At the follow up appointment, we review what happened with those goals. Did I reach them, or did I need a bit more time? Was it a realistic goal, or do we need to reassess and try something else?

My family also needs to know what's happening; it's not fair to keep them in the dark. My husband usually gets all the gory details, while my parents get enough to inform them but not so much that they worry. The information we share with our sons depends if we are close by or not. With us living in Vancouver and Mathieu living in Quebec, we try not to alarm him unless absolutely necessary and usually only give the "aftermath" to him and his family. With our youngest son, Ben, it's all he knows. He's had the misfortune of growing up with a chronically ill mom, so it's part of his normal world. We have seen some good come of it, though, as he's developed into a caring and compassionate young man who is great at noticing when I need help.

Even if you have the best, most understanding, most compassionate family and friends, there may still be times where they try to push you into something you can't do or give you questionable advice. Always try to remember that they do this because they care for you, and, when needed, do your best to keep them educated about your condition.

> **Journal reflection:** What are some ways to demonstrate grace?
>
> _____
>
> _____
>
> _____
>
> _____

Chapter 16

Alternative healing

June 11, 2016

Woke up and sat up in bed all by myself this morning. I stood up straight and wow, not too much pain! My back has not allowed me to do this in months! I went downstairs without complication. The pain is still there, but I am able to be completely upright instead of hunched over. It's an amazing feeling! I'm smiling and feeling the possibility that I could be healed, so long as I keep the faith that one day I will be healed. Today, with the encouragement of my dear friend Barb Wallick, I visited a women's wellness show. My first stop was with an angel card reader. She pulled out three arch angels. The first was Gabriel, the communicator. This indicated I would be successful at writing (the fact that she knew I was writing a book kind of freaked me out!), public speaking, and knowing how to accept and receive gifts from God. The second was

Michael, who represented courage and strength. This showed that what I was going through now would help me with my new success. The last one was Raphael, the healer. This meant that my healing would be my teaching tool for others. The angel card reader told me I would present a workshop with a five-step process; funny enough, I had just worked out the ADPIE "Nursing Process" (Assess, Diagnose/Determine, Plan, Implement, and Evaluate) care plan for myself. It's a five-step process I used to teach my nursing students; maybe this will be a workshop in the future for self-care!

The angel card reader said my soul knew I was coming today and was preparing me for messages I needed to receive. I was given such positive vibes and affirmations. She showed me how to change my words from something negative, such as "I have memory problems," to something more positive, such as "I'm improving my memory". I left feeling positive and hopeful. This could possible another amazing connection for healing myself—I've always had a thing for angels.

Although I'm Christian, I consider myself a very open-minded Christian. I believe that God gifts people with certain talents and insights to share with others.

My amazing friend Barb Wallick holds many titles; one of them is a chakra dance instructor. We've always teased each other about me being "Miss Science Nursey Christian" and her being "Miss Earth Airy Fairy," with nothing but respect of course. I tried her chakra dance session today, and it was surprisingly relaxing and very spiritual. I didn't feel weird or like people were staring at me, and I felt okay with the free, body-swaying movements. I moved on to another station at the wellness show for pulsed electromagnetic field (PEMF) cell stimulation. This was a magical magnetic mattress that you lay on for approximately fifteen minutes which creates a healing environment in the body. It actually reduced my back pain from a 9/10 to a 4/10. After an additional eight minutes, my left leg sciatic pain went down to 2/10.

Next, I tried a Reiki session. I could actually feel the energy from the practitioner's hands. She told me my some of my chakras were out of balance; my heart chakra was blocked and my crown chakra needed work. Although I wasn't sure what she meant at the time, I later did some research that clarified what she had told me. At the end of the treatment, I felt so relaxed—almost light and floaty, like I had just had a massage—and the reiki practitioner never even touched me! It was so lovely to feel so much peace. The therapy horses on site were also wonderful to see.

Am I convinced these alternative healing modalities are for me? I don't think there's a definitive answer here. For today, this is what I needed. I prayed God would open my heart to healing and that is what happened. I saw a glimpse of ME today—my old self, the one who loved to be happy.

There are a number of reasons why we choose what we choose to make us feel better. We choose to relieve physical, mental, or emotional pain. Sometimes, it's hard to tell which is worse. Personally, I think that emotional pain always feels harder to overcome. At least with physical pain there is usually something that will make it feel better. With emotional pain, there is not always an easy answer—it just takes more work and facing the problem head on.

In North America, there are standard methods of treatment used by almost every doctor. These include common treatments such as medications, physiotherapy, massage therapy, and counselling. However, these treatments are not always effective for everyone. For this reason, it's good to know that there are many alternative avenues of treatment available to you, not all of which your doctor will be knowledgeable about. Educating yourself on different treatment options is a great way to take control of managing your chronic illness. That being said, you should always discuss these treatments with your doctor before starting to make sure they are appropriate and safe for you.

Keep in mind, this is a never-ending process. Your illness is chronic; it's not going away, but symptoms can get better. We do have some control over managing how we feel. You can live with a better quality of life if you pay attention to what your body is telling you!

I'm currently taking five prescription medications for my lupus, fibromyalgia, osteoarthritis, migraines, anxiety, and neck, back, and hip pain. On a side note, one of the best people to consult about medication issues is your local pharmacist. He or she usually has the best and most up-to-date information regarding almost any kind of pharmaceutical. Even my own doctor has deferred occasionally to my pharmacist just in case. Having been a surgical nurse and an instructor, my knowledge on medication is quite substantial, but because I'm not teaching it every day like I used to, I'm a bit out of practice.

Below is a table that shows some of my go-to remedies, aside from using just prescriptions.

Diagnosis	Symptoms/complications	Treatment/prevention
Lupus	Muscles/joints pain	Water, CBD oil, Icy spray Heat/cold, Magnesium spray/tabs, MSM, Glucosamine.
	Fatigue	Water, Rest/lemon wter, Vit. C&D
	Yeast infections	Water, Probiotics/ topical cream, Candida diet, no sugar, no wheat.
	Mouth ulcers	Water, Liquid silver, Oragel, Oxygel.
Digestive disorder	Nausea	ginger Gravol, Pepto-Bismol chewable.
	constipation	Water, movement, stool softener.
Tendonitis, Bursitis	Elbow & forearm, Hip joint pain.	Water, CBC oil, Icy spray Heat/cold, Magnesium MSM, Glucosamine.
Sjogrens	Dry eye/leaky eye Dry Salivary glands	Renue eye drops "Biotene" rinse/ice
Hypertension	High blood pressure	Water, CBD oil
Asthma	Difficulty breathing	Breathing exercise
Eczema	Dry itchy skin	Water, Aveeno anti-itch lotion (triple oat complex)

Vertigo-Meniere's	Severe nausea & vomiting, imbalance, spinning room	Rest, dymenhydrante (full strength Gravol) Betahistadine
Kidney/bladder infections	Frequent urination, pain, difficulty urinating	Water, cranberry juice unsweetened

Note*** CBD oil is a sublingual marijuana oil without the high, see the section on medical marijuana

Essential oils are my favorite alternative treatment. I've used several different brands, from "Young Living" oils to "Sage," but a local aromatherapy shop called "TAP—True Aromatherapy Products & Spa" has always been one of my favorite healing places to visit. The atmosphere there is incredible. They welcome everyone—including our eighty-pound Goldendoodle "Cooper"—into the store. They provide herbal tea in delicate china teacups, free of charge, to enjoy while you peruse their offerings. TAP is filled with amazing oils, body and face mists ("Tranquil Water" and "Energy Mist" are my personal favourites), soaps, and lotions that come in a variety of calming fragrances. They have wonderful stones of amazing colours and, bonus, they offer spa services! I can't visit Fort Langley without going in; I always feel better after being in their positive vibe.

Different essential oils have different benefits, so I've included a list below of the uses for some of the types or combinations of oils. Always verify with your healthcare practitioner that these oils aren't contraindicated for your medical conditions or medications!

- Anxiety and stress: lavender, bergamot
- Exhaustion: rosemary and eucalyptus
- Fever: lemon, frankincense, peppermint

- Pain: copaiba lavender, peppermint
- Fibromyalgia: chamomile, lavender, marjoram
- Headaches, migraines, and sore muscles: peppermint and lavender
- Bruises, acne, dermatitis, eczema, and digestion: bergamot
- Asthma, nausea, sinus pain, digestion, inflammation: peppermint
- Congestion: lemon, eucalyptus, tea tree, peppermint
- Cold/flue: thieves and oregano
- Allergies: lavender, lemon, peppermint
- Cough, cleaner: lemon and thieves
- Vertigo, dizziness, nausea: helichrysum, lavender, lemon, and peppermint
- Ear infections, acne, antibacterial/antifungal, bug bites: tea tree
- Dry skin: frankincense (not too much if you have lupus, it boosts your immune system)

~

August 5, 2017

There has been research on how when we evoke thoughts of past pain, we then actually start feeling that physical or emotional pain again simply by remembering it. For me to be writing an entire book about living with both physical chronic pain and emotional pain and how it affected me has been more challenging than I thought it would be. I started having feelings of depression come out of nowhere, only to realise I knew exactly where it was coming from: the remembered pain. Even my body would start to feel achy and more tender than usual.

So, how do find a way to ease this pain while I'm writing? Enter the placebo effect. We've all heard of this effect, which is when a medication or treatment works because we believe that it will. This just proves the strong connection we have between our brain and our body. Can we feel better just by thinking positively? Wouldn't it be nice if we could save money by taking fake medication instead of relying on the ridiculously high-priced pharmaceutical industry?

There is also the effect of a caring ritual or treatment, which means that being cared for changes our perception of pain. There are some fairly complex scientific models of neurotransmitters in the middle frontal gyrus brain region and how the brain reacts to the placebo effect. However, since I'm not writing a biology paper, we will skip that part.

The takeaway message here is this: follow whatever medications or treatments your health practitioners have prescribed. Actively perform self-care habits such as eating healthy, sleeping well, meditating, exercising, and having an active social life. We can change our perception of pain by caring for ourselves. It can have the same neurological affect as a medication or treatment or a placebo medication for lessening symptoms. The placebo effect won't cure you, but it can change our perceptions of pain and our symptoms. However, this is not to say that this will replace any necessary medication; it's important to know that!

~

Chocolate or wine?

We all have vices; things we use for self-comfort. While they are not an official alternative treatment, indulging your vices—in moderation, of course—can give you that positive mental boost that you need. Sometimes they help you with your physical or emotional pain; sometimes, they just help you relax a little. So long as you don't become dependent on these vices, then they can be a great temporary pick-me-up.

One of my biggest vices is chocolate. Chocolate and I have a love hate relationship; I love chocolate, but it doesn't love me, or my hips for that matter. A good friend of mine claims that because chocolate comes from a bean, you can eat it whenever you want—it's really a salad! I continue to try to "encourage" our relationship, only in smaller portions than before. I buy the 70% dark chocolate made by Lindt and keep one bar in the fridge. That lasts me for an entire week, usually. This way I'm not overdoing it on the sweets, and dark chocolate comes with the bonus of containing antioxidants, so it's a healthier choice.

Another one of my vices is wine. Have you ever heard the phase, "Life's too short to drink bad wine?" I wholeheartedly agree. I keep a wine journal just to make sure no bad wine enters our home. Having a few pleasures in life is a good thing, and as you know moderation is what it's all about. With my medication moderation is key, meaning I don't drink very often. Wine is always good on a Friday night, or really any time during the week (after 5 p.m., of course). Generally, I try to limit myself to two glasses a week, which perfectly covers the weekend. I tend to only have a cold beer on weekends, if at all, and only if it won't interact with the medications I'm taking at the time.

"The Lord will fight for you; you need only to be still."
Exodus 14:14 (NIV)

Medical Marijuana

Over the past thirteen years, I have taken many different medications to control my systemic lupus, osteoarthritis, fibromyalgia, hypertension, and other ailments. Some have come and gone simply because they didn't work well, while others I've had severe reactions to and must avoid all together.

After a year of contemplation and discussions with my doctors, I applied for a license for medical marijuana through a recognized clinic and provider. My family doctor was honest enough to admit he hadn't been trained in the use of medical marijuana, which is why he was not comfortable with me using it to control pain and flare ups. Fair enough; at least he was being responsible in regard to his scope of practice. I did some of my own research—as I suggest everyone do with for a new modality of treatment, medication, or diagnostic test—and my GP and I reached an agreement to give it a try. We couldn't have imagined how effective it would be, or how quickly I would see benefits.

Before we go any further, I would like to remind you that this is my personal experience and should not be taken as medical advice. Wait until you have done your own research before you decide if it's right for you, and be knowledgeable about potential therapeutic uses, contraindications, adverse reactions, and so on. This important decision should be determined and agreed upon by you, your GP, and the Health Canada-approved agencies and suppliers.

The active ingredients that come from the marijuana plant are Tetrahydrocannabinol, more commonly known as THC, and Cannabidiol, otherwise known as CBD. THC has a quick onset and only last for a few hours, while CBD has a slow onset but will have a longer-lasting effect. The concentrations of these ingredients may vary depending on the strain of cannabis, and you can get isolated versions of these ingredients as well.

I won't speak too much about dosages or forms of medical marijuana such as oils, vaporizers, or edibles; my focus will solely be on communicating what is working for me. What I can tell you is that since I started taking CBD oil during the day and using a THC vaporizer before bed, my life has drastically changed for the better.

This is the first time in almost three years that I have been able to sleep through the night without waking due to pain and discomfort. That in itself is huge! I have also seen a decrease in my anxiety, my depression is not as doom-and-gloom as it once was, and the inflammation from my osteoarthritis has improved. I've also been able to stop taking my blood pressure medication because my heart rate has reduced to within the normal range, and I've been able to reduce my pain medications. For the longest time, I was up to six to eight Tylenol 3s per day! Now I typically only use one to two at most, unless I'm in a huge flare with major back spasms. My poor liver will not be as stressed as it once was by being inundated with so many different kinds of prescription drugs; I don't know how it has survived this long without major permanent damage!

The new-found advantage of my increased mobility is that it has given me back my independence! I haven't used my cane in almost eight months, and I'm walking on my own again. I can drive my own car again—unless I'm using THC—so I no longer have to rely on my husband, other family members, friends, and neighbors to drive me.

A few considerations about of medical marijuana

Is it pot?

What you call it is up to you. However, if you're wanting to steer away from stigma, use the medical terms such as medical cannabis, medicinal marijuana, THC, or CBD, depending on the strain of the plant/herb. There are different forms of cannabis, including smoking, vaping, oils, tinctures, orals/edibles, and topical ointments; all of these fall under the category of medical marijuana.

Go easy on your health care practitioner!

Chances are your family physician and/or specialist has received little to no formal training on medicinal marijuana. You have to work together as a team to decide if this is the right path for you and your health and well-being. Take some ownership; don't leave the burden of discovery to your GP. Get involved and do your own research by diving into credible resources on medical marijuana, such as Health Canada or the Journal of American Medical Association. Take your findings back to your GP so you can make a plan of action together.

What if your health care practitioner rejects the idea?

If your GP or health care practitioner is strongly against the concept of you using medicinal marijuana, don't take a simple "no" for an answer. Politely ask them why, but not before you come to them prepared with some answers of your own. I'd be willing to bet that they reject the idea due to lack of knowledge and experience. So, if you come prepared with backup resources to educate them, you may be able to further their knowledge on the subject.

Oh, I know what you're thinking. Isn't that what they get paid the big bucks for? Shouldn't they know this already? As a nurse, I can tell you there was absolutely none, nothing, zero, nada, diddly-squat information or training for nurses or doctors on medical marijuana during our primary training. The concept of using marijuana for medicinal purposes is in its infancy stages, and there are still so many contradictory positions that's not pharmaceutically mass-produced. Not to mention that there is a stigma attached to marijuana because of its only other purpose in the past was for recreational use to just get high.

What if my insurance won't cover the cost?

I can tell you firsthand that most insurance companies won't cover the cost of medicinal marijuana because it's still illegal in many parts of North America. However, in Canada you can apply for what is called "compassion pricing." When I retired from my Nursing career, I had no pension as my positions were considered part-time—even though I worked full-time hours—which left me with little to no benefits. Thankfully, the medical clinic where I received my prescription and the producer who grows the plants both gave me a disability discount. The clinic acts like a broker, providing the education and Physician for the legal prescription, and gives you recommendations for producers and suppliers recommended by Health Canada. I only had to provide documented proof that stated I am on a fixed disability income and submit a copy my Revenue Canada Tax return. After losing my Health Care Regional Coordinator paycheck, every little bit helps!

Know before you go- travel with Medical Cannabis

Local laws about possession, usage, and transportation of medical marijuana vary in all parts of North America. At the time of writing this book, in Canada you must carry a physician-signed prescription on your person along with the card from your certified supplier that proves you are legally allowed to carry and use medical marijuana. The Canadian Government is in the delicate process of legalizing marijuana, but currently the only form of legal marijuana is for medical purposes with the proper authorization.

Don't expect to cross through international boarders without potentially breaking the law. Ignorance is not bliss in this case! There are countries that carry very stiff penalties for marijuana possession and transport, even if it's for medicinal use. Find out in advance what the restrictions are before you land in jail abroad!

Not everyone needs to know!

One of my favorite quotes from Wayne Dyer is, "What other people think of me is none of my business!" Whether or not you decide to share with friends and family about your journey with medical marijuana, be prepared to know and understand your own beliefs first. The reasons why you have chosen to use medical marijuana is really no one's business but your own. I decided I wouldn't share my choice with anyone for a few months in order to give me time to feel comfortable with my own knowledge. With this approach, I then had the advantage of educating people accurately with confidence instead of being embarrassed and trying to flounder around with excuses.

Use it safely

DO NOT, under any circumstances, drive or make any important decisions while under the influence of cannabis or any other mind-altering medication. The CBD oil has no psychotic side effects, meaning there is no "high" or impairment, so it's alright to carry on as per usual. On the other hand, THC is quite potent and can cause extreme impairment of motor skills and cognition.

If you decide to try medical marijuana, as with any type of pain relief, start low and go slow! Make sure that you keep it safely stowed away from children and youth in your household, as is true for any and all medications. It also a good idea to have an open and honest conversation with any teens in the house about dangers of medications, including overdosing and potential life-threatening situations that can happen when you mess around with any kind of drug. You'll find some great information on the Health Canada website, or you can check with your local government for teen drug resources.

"And he sent them out to proclaim the kingdom of God and to heal the sick."
Luke 9:2 (NIV)

Journal reflection: What's one of your favorite ways to give yourself comfort? Why? Is it safe?

_____

_____

_____

_____

Chapter 17

Divine intervention and spirituality

For some of us, the word "spirituality" is followed by a question. What is it? Do I have it? If not, how do I get it? There are approximately fourteen definitions for the word and thousands of interpretations of what "spirituality" actually means.

One such interpretation comes from the Cambridge University Dictionary, which defines the term as follows: "The quality that involves deep feelings and beliefs of a religious nature, rather than the physical parts of life."

The word "spirituality" was originally associated with God, along with many competing religions and cultures. Some people argue that it is a separate experience from religion altogether, but all agree that it involves some form of a higher power. That power can come from your God or whomever that God may be; perhaps for you it is a rock, the ocean, a tree, or the universe. It doesn't matter. Spirituality is whatever you use to develop inner peace and a sense of your own wellbeing. Although there is no way to measure spirituality, some studies have shown that it is linked to health and wellbeing.

How did I use spirituality in my journey, you ask? I wouldn't have admitted this ten years ago, but I now connect my spirituality and healing with my faith as a Christian. Since I came to this realisation, I feel as though I've turned a corner in my healing. I owe a lot of it, if not all, to my faith in Christ. He was the only one I felt comfortable enough to turn to when I felt no one else would understand what I'm going through. Finding scripture that means something to you personally is so powerful and comforting. It's like having another parent available twenty-four seven. My parents are very supportive, but there were some things only God could hear; I didn't want to burden my parents with some of the darker times I'd suffered through.

I have a funny story of how I came to Christ. I wanted a sign from God that He was real, so I asked Him to show me HE was real. After I made that request, I noticed that every night when I came home from a meeting, there was either a hawk or an eagle in the exact same tree. Years later, when I was struggling, I would once again ask God to show me a sign He's was listening. Sure enough, there was my bird sitting in the same tree. On the days when I was not struggling, the tree was empty; I figure the bird was sitting in the tree of someone else who was more in need that day. Call it divine intervention or whatever you like; for me, it was an answer to prayer I will never forget. I owe most of my success to God and how He held me up during challenging times.

*"And whatever you do, whether in a word or deed, do it all in
the name of the Lord Jesus, giving thanks to God the Father
through him."*
Colossians 3:17 (NIV)

I wasn't always religious. My family didn't go to church
when I was growing up, so it wasn't something I felt I missed
out on. Once we had moved back to BC from living out East,
though, our lives became a bit more complicated, especially
after I was diagnosed with SLE.

As I discussed in a previous chapter, I went back to school
to become a nurse when Ben was four, and I faced a number
of extremely challenging times. It was a time when I felt very
alone and thought that I had to be in control. My identity
came from my career status and title as I was not brought up
with any type of faith.

Up to this point, any exposure I'd had to God made me feel
like I didn't belong or wasn't a good enough person because I
had not been baptized. I believed I was unworthy of prayer,
blessings, or the ability to have any connection to God. I heard
it once said that "you must ask for Gods help. You must initiate
the conversation." I did not relate or understand why this could
help anyone until we met Rod and Ainsley House. They were
our new neighbors upon returning to B.C. in 2003, and after
inviting us into their home they invited us to a more sacred
place: the Pacific Community Church. We attended a service,
and I felt welcome but out of place. I needed to find out what
I was missing out on; everyone seemed to be so connected to
some higher power, but I needed proof that Jesus was a real
human being that even non-Christian scientists could not
deny existed, not just some mythical character.

I jumped into an introductory group, then a Bible study,

a fashion show, and then a women's retreat. The experiences I had with other Christians and fellowship gave me real-life examples of how God was working in their lives. I wanted what they had: a relationship with a never-ending, loving, trusting Holy Spirit whom I could always count on. My "walk" had begun.

> *"For it is by grace you have been saved, through faith—and not that of yourselves, it is the gift of God—not by words, lest anyone should boast. We are God's workmanship, created in Christ Jesus to do good works, which God has prepared in advance for us to do."*
> **Ephesians 2:8-10 (NIV)**

A couple of years ago I bought a silver ring with the above-noted scripture engraved into the band to remind of me I'm not alone and that with my faith God is always there, in good times and in bad. I also gave an identical ring to one of my best friends, Danielle, who has been gracefully praying for me for years. It serves as a reminder that God is the higher power, not the medial world.

Then came 2005; it was a tough year. I was diagnosed with lupus, I had my first TIA, and Ben and I were in a car accident. We thought that my left arm had taken the brunt of the impact as it suddenly felt like it stopped working immediately after the crash; it just had no strength in it at all.

I was very sick and had no more fight in me. The stroke wasn't permanent, but I had difficulty pronouncing certain words for a while. It was almost like I had a sudden case of dyslexia when trying to read as the letters were all scrambled. I also had difficulty remembering words and couldn't finish sentences. I was even spelling my own name wrong.

There was speculation in the medical world that my lifespan could be cut short if this attack on my brain were to happen again. Would my two-year-old son possibly have to grow up without his mother? I wanted to be prepared and protect my family just in case, but I didn't know how. I was angry with God for yet again testing my strength, especially after all the commitment I had put into finding Him. Why wasn't He helping me? Suddenly, I realized that I had forgotten to actually ask Him for help.

I literally went down on the floor on my hands and knees started yelling at God, "Okay, I get it! I do not have control. My life is in your hands. Please help me, do what you need to do." I was trying something I had never done before, and it was a very difficult thing to do with my Type A personality. I had to completely trust my entire future to someone else.

"But we rejoice in our sufferings, because we know that suffering produces perseverance; perseverance, character; and character, hope. And hope does not disappoint us, because God poured out His love into our hearts by the Holy Spirit."
Romans 5:3-5 (NIV)

From then on, I started to pray or have conversations with God, which can also be a form of meditation. Slowly, with lots of prayer and the help of wonderful friends, family, neighbours, and my church family, I began to feel there was hope. I started to regain my strength and finally went into remission that fall, although a few short months later I was back in a flare up that lasted two years. It was certainly God who healed my heart and my mind, and then my body followed. So, there's my answer: Christ was healing me because I truly believed he could, and he did.

I publicly pronounced my life to Jesus in April of 2006. I decided I need to be fully committed, and therefore I that needed to be baptized. When the big day approached, I was nervous and excited! I was baptized in my blue Nike T-shirt and shorts by our good friend Pastor Jim in a tub of very cold water. It was such a transformation to become a child of Christ. We feel so blessed to still be part of this church family.

I now have a better view of how God sees me. I know that when I pray, He hears me. He doesn't always answer, and for good reason. His plans or schedule are not up to us, so we must simply have faith in Him. His plan is better than any plan you could have for yourself, and I can't wait to see what he has in store for me.

We're not always at church on Sundays; in fact, it's been a good two years since we attended regularly. It's mostly because I haven't been able to sit for too long, or because getting out of bed and getting dressed before 9 a.m. was too painful and difficult. Other times I was just not up to answering all the questions about why I had to walk with a cane.

Even though we don't go to church often, I know our church family continues to pray for us as we do for them. Two of my prayer warriors, Shelley and Ainsley, always keep me in their prayers, and I know God has used both of them to connect me to Him. I also know that the next battle against this autoimmune disease will be backed by the hand of our creator Christ. This is whom I will commit my life and my future to.

"Trust in the Lord with all your heart and lean not on your own understanding; in all your ways acknowledge Him, and He will make your paths straight."
Proverbs 3:5-6 (NIV)

While my spirituality is mostly centered around my relationship with God, I do enjoy other aspects of spirituality in nature. The beautiful tall trees that provide us shade and colour in the fall, the flowers that encourage new life in the spring, the crystal-clear water flowing in a river or the crisp white caps on the waves of the Pacific Ocean; they all add to my spirituality and sense of wellbeing. I often go into nature for healing. There is a practice in Japan called Shinrin-yoku, which is described as "the act of walking in a forest and actively breathing the air." This act of forest bathing is supposed to help reduce stress including lower your blood pressure, your heart rate. It certainly has been a major stress reducer for me.

> *"Your word is a lamp to my feet and light to my path."*
> **Psalm 119:105 (NIV)**

The mind, body, and spirit connection

I see the mind, body, and spirit as a pyramid, much like Maslow's hierarchy of needs. This is a theory where a person's needs are placed in a pyramid, with the most fundamental needs at the bottom. From the bottom to the top, Maslow separates our needs into physiological needs (such as sleeping and eating), safety, love/belonging, esteem, and self-actualization. The difference is that I see spirituality as my foundation. The mind can only handle so much stress, and then it transfers the stress and anxiety over to the body. This we then see as physical symptoms such as headaches, body malaise, fatigue, insomnia, and restlessness, as well as emotional signs such as agitation, inability to make decisions, confusion, and depression to name a few.

After my mind and body gave in to disease and pain, my

spirit was finally broken. Once that spirit is broken, it's a long, hard, and lonely road back to finding solid ground again. My faith has taught me to listen to what God is trying to tell me or to pay attention to the people God has put in my path; there is a reason they have entered my life at the time that they did. There have been many instances when I thought there was no one I could turn to except God because I was too embarrassed to admit I couldn't handle fighting this all on my own. All I had to do was to pray and ask for help, and it would come in some form or another. Sometimes it would take longer than I had wanted but, it would come.

"For I know the plans I have for you, declares the Lord, plans to prosper you and not harm you, plans to give you hope and a future."
Jerimiah 29:11 (NIV)

So now we to swing back towards the other side of my beliefs, and that's science. I love that there is so much agreed-upon acknowledgment on the subject of the scientific connection between body, mind, spirituality, and soul. It is truly amazing how interconnected our physical being is with our spiritual being. I fight pain every day and will have systemic lupus for the rest of my life; there is no cure for this potentially life-threatening disease. Is there a chance to live with a good quality of life and less symptoms though? I believe there is.

While my faith is important to my healing process, so is the knowledge that our brain becomes conditioned from being in constant pain to keep sending the same repeated pain signals to our body. This raises the question, "How much control do we have over pain?" There have been many studies and theories on how we can control our own pain simply by re-wiring the signals we send to our brain. If we focus on being in pain all the time, we will be in pain all the time. If we can somehow focus on gratitude and what we can do to change our situation, it changes the pain receptor patterns we use to communicate in our brain and we experience a more positive outcome. That's not to say that we will no longer experience pain; instead, it means that we have the ability within ourselves to decrease our heightened pain signals through positive messages that release our "happy hormones," such as endorphins. The more positive we feel, the less prominent our pain is. Hence the term "laughter is the best medicine"!

So, how do we do this re-wiring or reprogramming? Well, because the body and mind are connected, we can actually condition our brain to be less sensitive to remembered pain receptors by paying attention to our fight-or-flight response to pain. For example, if I'm afraid of being in pain and stop myself from participating in an activity, the signal I'm sending is fear-based. The stress response to the stimuli (activity) is to stop doing that activity. This response sends a warning signal to allow the brain to tell us that this activity causes pain. Eventually, every time I try that activity I will feel pain, because my brain has repeatedly been conditioned to do so. The more I condition my brain to feel pain, the faster the pain will come on. This is what chronic pain is. Dr. Lorimer Moseley, an Australian Pain Scientist, describes chronic pain as follows: "As your time living with pain increases, the involvement of the tissues reduces and the involvement of the nervous system increases." In other words, as time passes we condition our brain to fear the pain and thus engage our brain to remember the pain, which delays healing.

"Whether you think you can, or you can't, you're right."
Unknown

If my response to stress is that of a more positive mind set, I'm less likely to experience remembered pain. The reverse is also true. This is particularly common with fibromyalgia patients. The more depressed I got, the worse my pain and immobility got. This is where counselling, psychological assistance, and timeline therapy can be beneficial to chronic pain patients. This is not to say that the pain is in your head; but, it *is* in your brain. It's not your fault, it's the process of our central and peripheral nervous system and how they receive and send signals to and from our brain. The good news is that we have the power to change it!

There is a difference between actual physical tissue damage and remembered pain. Obviously physical tissue damage, such as a broken leg or bulging discs in your vertebrae, need proper medical care as well as a positive belief system. Remembered pain, though, mostly requires that reprogramming. Once I started my gratitude journal, meditation, prayer, and visualizing myself as being healthy again, I started experiencing moments of lowered pain. Timeline therapy and creating a vision board were also a tremendous help as they allowed me to release past negative beliefs about myself, regain my confidence, and move forward in a positive path of self-love.

Pain medication has been a big part of my life for the past fourteen years, but after creating a more positive outlook on my life situation, I'm happy to say that I've been walking again with no cane for eight months now. It's also allowed me to significantly reduce the amount of pain medication I need. I'm almost certain I would not have been able to make this improvement without positively retraining my brain and creating more endorphins and happier experiences.

> **Journal reflection:** If you or a loved one has a chronic illness, can you imagine life if they got better? What does it look like?
>
> _____
>
> _____
>
> _____
>
> _____

Chapter 18

Celebrate, grieve and celebrate again!

June 27, 2016

I found out from my GP that my Rapid Access to the Spinal Clinic was rejected. Apparently, my back isn't bad enough for me to be seen by their doctors, and I need just a bit more damage to my spine to qualify as an "urgent or surgical needs" patient. I would have to wait another eight months to see the Neurosurgeon, at which point he would decide if I'm a candidate for back surgery or not. I don't want to have back surgery; in fact, I'd like to avoid it all costs. But I do want some answers.

Where do we go from here? How long will I suffer with this pain? Will I ever be able to walk like a normal forty-something-year-old again? I'm unable to drive, sitting is almost impossible, and sleeping, um, what is sleeping again? So here we go, back to the drawing board so to speak.

When I finally met with the neurosurgeon, he told me there's not much they could do for now and that surgery would not be recommended. This is great news! However, I couldn't help but feel frustrated that we still didn't have a definitive answer as to what was causing my severe back, neck, and hip pain. We may have to live with the impending doom of another possible diagnosis that had been a suspected for a while: Ankylosing Spondylitis. This condition is roughly described as the spine fusing together, straightening and restricting movement in my neck and back. My range of motion is already limited, which has prevented me from driving as I can't perform the necessary shoulder checks. I can feel my life taking a turn we weren't expecting, one where my independence would again become less and less.

I keep telling myself that just because the genetic disease markers are showing up in the blood work didn't mean that the diagnosis is confirmed. The medical imaging so far was not conclusive, so what's the answer? We may have to live with the fact that there is no answer, just more questions.

They have given me the option of having more Fluoroscopy injections in my SI joints. This is the joint at your pelvis, connecting to your sacrum near base of your spine, and when it is damaged or pinched the SI nerve can send extremely painful electric-like shocks from the base of your spine down the back of your thigh and all the way down to the foot. It can be literally paralyzing. I have this issue on both sides. Lucky me...not!

The injections are less than pleasant. First, they numb the sacroiliac joint with local anesthetic, and then they put a four-inch lumbar needle into the joint and inject a contrast dye so they can ensure that the needle is placed properly and that medication is distributed correctly. Oh, and don't sneeze, cough, fart, or make any kind of movement; there is a four-inch needle sticking into your back! You know how when you leave the dentist, your mouth is frozen and you can't feel the side of your face? You feel like that after this procedure, only it's your bum that's frozen so you kind of have a noodle leg until the anesthetic wears off.

My next fluoroscopy appointment is at a rapid access overflow clinic on July 19th . It's only about a month away, but it can't come fast enough! I've been spending a lot more time with my friend, Hugo, which is the name I've given my cane. I've also put on a lot of weight, which is unfortunately a common side effect of using Corticosteroid drugs. They are a necessary evil in trying to get better, although when you first take them they tend to make it feel like you're getting worse.

Due to cardiovascular complications, my feet are now swelling more and more every day. If your heart is not cooperating, the fluid tends to pool in the legs and drain down into the feet. This makes it painful to walk or stand for too long. The lupus has attacked my heart a few times, causing my blood pressure to increase significantly. This has increased the amount of stress on my heart, which creates another condition called left ventricular hypertrophy. In other words, my heart has slightly enlarged because of all the pressure it's under.

Aside from all that, I'm more concerned with how I look. It sounds shallow, I know, but I just don't recognize the person looking back at me in the mirror. I know the weight gain is from the medication, my back, and my hips, but I've never been this overweight before in my life. It's almost impossible to exercise because of my immobility; every step I take sends stabbing sharp knives in my lower spine. Who is this crippled, sick, bloated, weak person? Where did I go?

I'm feeling anxious as my retirement party is coming up on July 23rd and we are going to visit François' family in Montreal in August. I don't want to be seen like this.

~

July 15, 2016

It's my birthday! No big deal, right? Actually, it is a huge deal. Years ago, patients that were diagnosed with systemic lupus alone were given a five- to ten-year survival rate after their initial diagnosis. I have surpassed my expiry date!! So, I celebrate that I get to celebrate another year and another birthday!

Some people dread getting older, but I consider it a privilege that not everyone gets to experience. My son Ben was working in our townhouse complex through a youth program we've had here every summer for about three to four years now. This morning he left me a note that said, "I can't make you breakfast cause I had to work, so here's a birthday banana!" So sweet! What a precious and thoughtful gift; those are my favorite!

Is there a better way to spend your birthday than out shopping? Not for me! I don't get out much on my own these days because of my mobility, but today is a good pain day so here I go. I head to a Michael's craft store to look for cotton yarn. I've taken up crochet since I've been on sick leave as I needed to have a hobby to keep my brain busy. I also have osteoarthritis in my hands, so I can only do so much crochet before my hand goes numb. While the work is stop and go, I still get to produce something beautiful. My latest project is making cotton dishcloths; they were a big hit last Christmas, so I am making more for family and friends. I love that I can still bring joy to others. I love that I can create things with my hands and feel a sense of added purpose.

Tonight, I will continue the celebrations with some of my "tribe" girlfriends at the local pub. These are the some of the most important women in my life. You know the ones you can call at 3 a.m. to help you go and hide the body? I'm kidding, but you get my point. They're also the same incredible women that have taken care of my child at a moment's notice when I'm being rushed to the hospital. Ains and Lou, you're the best!

I must rest up so I can go out for dinner. I nap more frequently now. At forty-six, having to have a nap during the day seems crazy, but it really helps with the chronic fatigue and stress levels. This in turn helps to lower my pain as well. My hair looks great, I've got a cute outfit on, and off I go to celebrate at the pub. I won't last long, but I will enjoy every bit of it, along with my peach tea and bourbon! I know what you're thinking: why would I be having alcohol with all this medication and inflammation? Well, it's my birthday dammit! I'm having a cocktail!

François came home with a helium balloon, which makes the celebration seem even more legit! I'm grateful today for getting to live and celebrate another year. I'm blessed to have so many wonderful friends who love me and are still hanging around. I'm also grateful for self-tanner, because I just feel better with a bit of glow about me. Feeling loved and beautiful!

By the way, my retirement party was amazing! So many wonderful friends, family, former colleagues, and students were there to wish me well. My husband presented me with a beautiful yellow topaz ring set in white gold and said that "in sickness and in health, he would spend the rest of his life beside me." There wasn't dry eye in the room!

~

Don't forget to play

When you're in a constant state of debilitating pain, it's a struggle to be a positive person all on your own. I highly recommend that you purposefully engage yourself in as much fun as much as possible!

My husband is an avid biker, both pedal and motor, which is not something I'm able to enjoy often. I find being on a bike can be a painful experience. "How can you not be comfortable on a bike," François will ask me. "Pretty fricking easily," I'll respond! Having my arms outstretched into one position for more than a few minutes is extremely painful for my wrists and my shoulders. Sitting for an indefinite amount of time on anything, never mind a tiny bike seat, hurts my back and my butt.

However, I like to spend time with François, and if bicycling is the best way to do that so be it. In order to make this possible, I had to get a new bike that would be easier on my body. I wanted something fun but comfortable, so I got a pretty, butter-yellow bike with a cute little bell! It has no bar to climb over, which made it much easier to get on and off; I won't have to injure myself just getting on. I would, however, be really good at hurting myself getting off.

One day, we were out on a short ride through the neighborhood and I was showing off how fast I could go. I passed both of the boys and was coming to a bit of a hill. I thought this would be a great time to slow down and wait for them, which would also give me a chance to catch my breath. I put my foot out to catch the curb while at the same time putting all my weight onto that side of the bike. Unfortunately,

I shifted my weight too much and missed my footing, and the whole bike flipped over on top of me. I ended up upside-down, with my pretty yellow bike tangled with my legs, while my hip and elbow crashed into the ground. Yes, I had a helmet on, but what I should have had on was hockey gear! François and Ben love this story, so at least I made them laugh, right?

It's important to laugh at yourself

You have to be able to laugh at yourself, even in times of pain; if we can't see the humour in things that are painful, we won't survive. Far too often, we only pay attention to how horrible things can be, but there's a humorous side to almost every situation.

For example, I've had many days where my legs are unstable, which causes me to trip or lose my balance and fall over. My family thinks it's quite hilarious, so instead of helping me up François and Ben will be in stiches watching me flounder and wiggle on the ground. Don't worry, they do eventually help me up. It must look pretty funny though, because they'll still be laughing about it hours later. I wasn't laughing at first, but then I couldn't help myself. I'm sure if we sent footage into America's Funniest Home Videos, I'd be worth a few bucks!

While were talking about being silly, our dog gives us so much joy. Our spazzy Goldendoodle Cooper expresses the purest sense of joy when he gets his ball. I want that simple pure happiness of having my most favourite thing in the world and having fun with my family.

What is my ball of joy? I feel joy when I feel God's presence in my life. I also feel joy when I'm creating things or being in nature. When my body is cooperating, we go for walks. If not, I find things at home to keep my creative side busy, whether it's moving the artwork around to different rooms in the house or changing the bedding for each season. Yes, I am that person that has different linens and window treatments for each season! I'm also a serial dishcloth crocheter, if that's even a word. I haven't done anything more complicated yet, other than the odd scarf, toque, or Christmas ornament. I have been known to pull a ball of yarn out my purse at Ben's hockey games or practices, the doctor's office, and on car rides; I have my newest crochet project at the ready just about anywhere, anytime.

Learn to celebrate and enjoy the good times to help get you through the bad ones.

"May the God of hope fill you with all joy and peace as you trust in him, so that you may overflow with hope by the power of the Holy Spirit."
Romans 15:13 (NIV)

Journal reflection: What can you celebrate about your life?

_____

_____

_____

_____

Chapter 19

It takes a village

If you've ever been really ill and haven't been able to participate in something you wanted to do, you've surely felt left out. After twelve years of missing out on family events, friends' birthday celebrations, Christmas parties, charity fundraisers, my son's hockey games, days at the beach, family reunions, and so on, you'd think I'd be used to it by now. However, this is not the case. I still feel guilty for not be able to go to that party or meet girlfriends for dinner; even being unable to walk the dog gives me a terrible feeling of hopelessness.

There are so many who don't understand what it's like to live with a chronic illness that isn't visible to the outside world. Mine is severe crippling pain that a least a few times a month prevents me from walking. Other times it the debilitating depression that sneaks up on me after battling a flare up where yet again I feel I'm being judged, because I was able to do groceries one day and unable to get out of bed the next.

Rejection is something no one likes to face. It's like reliving those horribly embarrassing high school nightmares over and over. Like imagining a time when you're the only one that isn't in on the joke, only to discover the joke is on you and every is staring at you in disbelief and whispering about you, trying to get away from you as quickly as they can.

One great first step to get past these feelings of exclusion and rejection is to find groups of like-minded people that you can join. For example, I've been attending a few women's events in the past two to three years. I've walked into the event with a cane, forty to fifty pounds overweight, with different autoimmune diseases. I felt embarrassed, but I was inspired by the amazing women I met, many whom I'm happy to say are now great friends! Can I actually change my life like these other women had? Can I get my curvy, healthy, athletic body back? Can I get back my love for life and have laughter as my everyday medicine, instead of the twelve-plus pills a day I'm taking now? I think I can. I also network with others who have a similar condition to mine, so I can glean any new info from them.

I also have dear friend that participates with an organization called the British Columbia Mobility Opportunities Society, which is a not-for-profit organization that enables people with disabilities to experience great outdoor activities like hiking on a Trail rider (an alternative all-terrain wheelchair) mobilized by volunteers. I was amazed when I saw the photos. Now there's no excuse not to enjoy beautiful BC!

That feeling of inclusion and acceptance doesn't always come from friends; it can even come from complete strangers. One Sunday, my family and I visited the lovely Fort Langley and happened to stumble upon a shop called Wild Moon & Star studio art. It's a whimsical shop filled with amazing handcrafted gifts made from silver, glass, and gemstone. I was just finishing this book when I met the wonderful owner, who—after hearing my story—chose to gift me with a healing crystal of clear quartz. She then blessed both myself and the crystal. I was amazed by her genuine intuition to know how much it would mean to me, especially as I was going through a pivotal time in my life. My mother was with me to witness this spiritual moment, and she bought me a lovely hand-crafted bowl entitled "Tidal bowl" to house my new crystal. What a special day! I was left floating in hope and gratitude for all these experiences given to me. Love and light, baby, love and light!

~

July 20, 2016

Today was reserved for shopping with my dear friend's daughter, who I will refer to as K. It's her nineteenth birthday today. If there was any advice I'd give on friendship, it's this: nurture the relationships that love you back. You'll get so much more out of them. It does take some effort, except for the "being there for each other" part; this is easily done when you care deeply about the other person—and them about you—and you enjoy spending time with them. My friend, who I will call A, and I have been friends since 2003. When we met, our kids were still in diapers. We both were in the throes of motherhood and shared so many of the same problems, so the friendship just came easy. Why? Because we took care of each other. I would watch her kids, and she would watch mine. There were shared carpools to summer camp, church, and hockey practice. A was also present at the beginning stages of my lupus diagnosis in 2005, and she was there for me during this scary and uncertain time in our lives. We've become the surrogate mother to each other's children. Our kids grew up together and know and love us like family.

So, my shopping date with K was cut short this morning by not one, not two, but three urgent phone calls—one from my cardiologist and two from my GP—to get to the emergency department of the nearest hospital as soon as humanly possible. I called my GP's office and my doctor was away, but his locum (substitute doctor) wanted to see me before I went to the hospital. While I'm on my way to the doctor's office, I prayed to God and gave control to Him. I was bracing myself for the worst, but after I released the responsibility of controlling the situation, an incredible sense of peace came over me. I never once felt sad or scared; I just knew He would do His job and I had no control in any way, other than to tell my body to surrender to God and His will. I rushed to my GPs office and was immediately taken in. Our meeting was short and sweet. The doctor's question to me was, "When did you have your last heart attack?" I'm thrown off by this question because I've never had a heart attack! Oh wait, except for this one time about a month earlier, when we were up at Whistler for Ben's Provincial High school band competition.

Ben plays trombone in his senior high school's Concert Band. Every spring there is a Provincial Music competition called the Cantando up in beautiful Whistler, BC. This was his first year competing, so we were very excited for him and his band mates. The weather was sunny and warm enough for shorts and our hotel was right in the village—great for walking to all the shops and restaurants, and all the competition venues were close by.

I started having chest pain. This is a symptom I've

had in the past—usually brought on by a condition called costochondritis, which is inflammation in between the ribs that causes sharp, shooting pain when you inhale—so we weren't too concerned. Usually the pain only lasts for a few seconds and goes away with stretching and breathing exercises. This time, however, the pain got more intense and breathing was becoming difficult. I told François what was happening. He wasn't worried; as I said, this happens at least once every other week or so. But then my jaw started to hurt and sweating and nausea followed. If you didn't already know, these are all classic signs and symptoms most women feel with the onset of a heart attack. Women typically experience chest pain with jaw and neck pain, versus men who experience arm and chest pain. Both men and women can have the shortness of breath, sweating, and nausea.

Now I start to panic. Am I having a friggin' heart attack? I knew I needed to calm down. I had François get me some 81-milligram aspirin in case it was a heart attack, and I chewed four tabs to make sure the bloodlines kept moving. After laying down for about hour, the chest pain subsided but I was still feeling a bit weak. However, because I'm a nurse, everyone looks to me fix the situation and give the all-clear so we can move on. As a result, I tend to minimize the severity of any symptoms I feel. What we should have done is gone to the hospital ASAP, or better yet called an ambulance, but instead we went on with our day. I also didn't bother going to the hospital because there have been too many times that I've gone to emergency only to be sent home because they could find anything. Shame on me; this wasn't a smart decision. Overlooking what happened was a big mistake on my part.

After this event, everyone decided to go shopping and I chose to tag along. After all, when one is in Whistler, one must go shopping! The pain seemed to have subsided for now but I was still feeling very short of breath. As per usual, I ignored it and went on with my day. It is my way of dealing with my pain issues. I try not to make it anyone else's problem, because it can be so disruptive.

Back to the present day. The bloodwork my cardiologist had previously ordered had come back, and one of the tests had shown that I had experienced a recent cardiac trauma. Needless to say, the clinic staff were in a panic. They didn't want to take any chances, so they sent me to the hospital with a hand-written note from the doctor that I'm to been seen immediately and tested for a pulmonary embolism (a blood clot in the lung) or a deep vein thrombosis (a blood clot in the lower extremities, usually in the legs).

Time was critical; my life could be in imminent danger. I called François at work and told him the situation and that he needed to meet me at home and then drive me to the hospital. In hindsight, it would have made more sense to just meet him there or to have him pick me up at the doctor's office as I probably should not have been driving at this point. We met at home and left a note for Ben that I was just going to the hospital for some tests, with no mention as to the seriousness of the situation. As mothers, we protect our kids from so many things that they don't need to know or are not old enough to understand. I never thought I'd be hiding my illnesses in order to comfort others and not bring them any undue distress, but here I was.

After checking in at emergency, I'm rushed through the long line right to the front because of the urgency of my cardiac crisis. The nurses at the registration are baffled and confused by my situation because I'm only forty-six. They don't seem to know what lupus is, and being a teacher I launch into my "autoimmune disease" tutorial. They are amazed that I don't seem to be in any distress considering all I have to deal with; I've always been told I present well as a patient, which isn't always a good thing when you have invisible illnesses or pain. I informed them about the systemic lupus, osteoarthritis, fibromyalgia, lymphangiomyomatosis, Sjogrens, Renaud's, granuloma annulare, bulging discs in my spine, and the degenerative condition of my neck. There's more, but you get the idea. Then comes the "**you don't look sick**." If I had a dollar for every time I've heard that phrase, I'd be a cagillionaire.

I'm fast-tracked to triage and there's a scramble of nurses putting in an IV, giving me oxygen, and doing vital signs—blood pressure, heart rate, and respirations. The lumbar SI injection that I was given yesterday was getting quite tender, so I asked my nurse if she could get me some pain relief. I've been receiving four-and-a-half inch lumbar needles into my sacroiliac joints every three months, which help reduce my pain so I can walk. While all of this is going in, I'm thinking, *I really don't have time to be sick*; my retirement party was in a few days and I had so much to do still. Oh well, the hospital was the right place for me to be so I could be tested and treated and have other people take care of me.

They sent me off for a chest x-ray, then a CT contrast for my lungs, and finally a Doppler ultrasound on my right calf, all checking to see if there's a potentially life-threatening blood clot in either my lungs or my leg. If you've never had a contrast dye by IV, it feels like your peeing your pants! I was lucky enough that the staff were able to fast-track me into my own cubicle instead of waiting with the rest of the sick people in emergency. There I spent the day with François. My poor husband, he was so worried.

We were so grateful to neighbours who fed our son dinner that night. There were lots of phone calls and texts to family to keep them updated. We had lost one our beloved uncles the week before, so emotions were already running high.

We wait for doctor to give us my diagnosis. The clock just seems to go slower by the minute. I start deciding what François will need to get for me from home should I indeed be admitted to the hospital for treatment or observation.

Finally, after a long day of diagnostic tests and blood work, the doctor finally came with news. Some kind of anomaly around the lungs had shown up on the CT scan; in fact, I was actually suffering from a pleuritic attack. This is an increase in the fluid around the outer lining of the lungs, which can cause a similar tightness of the chest, laboured breathing, pain, and nausea as one would feel during a heart attack. At the time they suspected it was caused by either an infection somewhere or some sort of lupus flare up. My blood test had been seriously off the charts, which had given the appearance of a heart attack, but apparently this can happen with lupus patients. Aren't I lucky! The doctor also noted that it could be a progression of my lymphangiomyomatosis (LAM), a condition that causes cysts to grow in my lungs. He said the cysts appeared to be larger and had multiplied, possibly causing some shortness of breath, but that this was not the main concern for now. They gave me some pain medication, and then I was released home to bed rest.

～

While this was not a heart attack, my situation still could have been dangerous. If my breathing had become too laboured, I could have suffered a collapsed lung. The pleuritic attack also could have been the result of some kind of infection, which I'm prone to because of the immunosuppressive medication I take every day. This medication is a double-edged sword: it stops my autoimmune system from attacking my body and organs, but it lowers my immune system so I'm a sitting duck for infections.

Despite the urgency and scariness of the day, I felt loved and cared for by everyone involved. Although I spent the day in the hospital, I was where I was supposed to be and there were people taking care of me. I had a village of support—the neighbours who watched my kids, the hospitals staff who took care of me, my family who checked in on me, and my husband who stayed with me and kept me company—and it made all the difference in the world.

Know your tribe

There are days when you feel like the whole world is against you. I've learned very quickly who I can trust, who I can really on, and who has truly been there for me. I grieve for the friendships that I no longer qualify to be a part of. I don't fit their lifestyle anymore; I'm not the same outgoing athlete I once was. I see my old friends and colleagues on Facebook with their healthy, shining bodies and their seemingly perfect lives, posting pictures of themselves running "tough mudder" or "colour me rad" races. I'm angry and I'm jealous because I want to do what they're doing, and my brain can't understand why they are allowed to do this and I'm not. My version of tough mudder is getting out of bed in the morning.

I've lost many friends along this journey. Some are afraid, while others may think I'm putting on an act and believe I should just try harder. The few that remain are my life preservers that keep me afloat when I feel like I'm drowning. I would not have survived without Christ as my captain and my friends as his faithful sailors. Not that family isn't important or special, but they don't get to choose you. Our friends make the decision to stay with us, not because of blood but because of a chosen love for us.

Maintaining friendships is difficult, and if you are chronically ill you may not always able to follow through on commitments. I'm not the reliable rock I used to be, and it hurts me. I'm so glad I have kind, caring, and genuinely compassionate women in my life that don't make me feel guilty for not always being well.

So, here's my shout out to the powerful and loving women in my life. You know who you are! I won't name names, because I know I'll forget someone. Some of you are childhood or school friends, some of you are neighbors, and some of you are new friends. I love you all more than you know, and I thank you with all my being and spirit. I could never have made it this far without your encouragement, babysitting, transportation, meals, gifts, yoga, kindness, forgiveness, and most of all, your prayers. Thank you, my earth angels!

Journal reflection: Who's in your tribe? Do you nurture those relationships?

_____

_____

_____

_____

Chapter 20

At the end of the day

"The Lord will fulfill His purpose for me".
Psalm 138:8 (NIV)

July 5, 2017

My conference call today with my publisher was supposed to be an update on the status of my manuscript. I'm in a panic as I haven't gotten as far as I would have liked. I'm avoiding my computer and making excuses about other things I "need" to do because the thought of writing down all the stories of the past twelve years of pain, trauma, surgeries, diagnostic testing, changing doctors, and dealing with social isolation and fear of judgment terrifies me. I feel like I'm reliving all the emotions just from reading my journal notes. I need to remember the reason I started writing this book in the first place: to help others with chronic illness. Thank God I'm not alone. You are not alone.

Try to be patient with yourself. Your body is trying to tell you that it needs to be taken care of. If it's reacting in a negative or painful way and symptoms are flaring up, that's a signal to stop and rest and reassess where to go from here. Frustration leads to pain, pain leads to mental anguish, and then the winding rugged road of depression lies ahead. This is all normal, so take the time you need. It doesn't matter how long you've been at this battle; some days, it still gets the better of you. My pain and illnesses have no regard for my training in Disaster Response and Critical Incident Stress Management. Nor do my pain or illnesses care that I'm an experienced Surgical Nurse used to facing stress, emergencies, and even death in the workplace on a daily basis. My pain and illnesses ignore the fact that I was a leader in Health Care Education and a well-respected member of the Health Care and Education societies.

Chronic pain and illness are a rollercoaster of emotion, and unfortunately this is true no matter how educated or experienced you are. You're human, not God. Only He knows why you're going through this. It doesn't have to make sense now, so learn to be okay with not knowing why. Stop getting in your own way and let God do His job. Be grateful to your body for letting you know you have limitations. Respect your body for what it does for you instead of focusing on what it doesn't do.

Your body sends us signals not to upset us, but to warn us that something is wrong. Be thankful we were created with such a wonderful security system. Although faulty at times, our body's defence mechanism is usually on target.

Sometimes a method of treatment or medication that's been working for the past five years no longer works for you; some medications can actually become toxic to your body over time. If so, it will tell you by way of signs and symptoms. I've had to change my blood pressure medication three times over the past few years, simply because my body decided it didn't like that treatment anymore. So, if your body is showing negative side effects from treatments or medication or even the environment, your need to speak with your doctor. You may only need a simple dosage adjustment, or you might have to do a complete stoppage of the drug or treatment

Be patient and kind to your body and your mind. Don't push yourself because you think, "I can do this, I've been through this before, I can handle it!" Promise yourself this: stop pushing so hard, and stop having ridiculous expectations that you can "tough it out." Allow yourself to time to rest up if you need it. If there was ever anyone who understands this, it's me.

It's okay to not be okay.

~

Dec 28, 2017

Today I'm having trouble seeing the light or good in my life. I watched way too much TV yesterday and ate unhealthy sugary foods, which was followed by regret. I couldn't get dressed until 4:30 p.m.

Times like these always seem all-consuming, leaving me feeling as if I have no control over what my brain is thinking or what I can do. Why do I feel so paralyzed? What is holding me back?

Where do I draw the line between rest and lifelessness?

How did I get like this today? Was it the rain washing away the snow? Was it the fact that Christmas is now over, and I feel like I was robbed some of the joy of the season because of my stupid hospital stay? Was it because when I suggested we go snowshoeing yesterday, my husband said I couldn't do things like this anymore? Was that it?

I feel paralyzed that my book is this heavy project that will never get done, but I have to be done in a few weeks. I don't know what I will do after this book. I don't think I want to run a business, but I'm not sure I can survive without a career. It seems like I was crossing this same bridge exactly a year ago and thinking the same negative, self-destructive thoughts. That I don't have anything to look forward to. Am I happy without a title? Do I miss being a nurse, or do I miss *saying* I'm a nurse? In truth it's both, but I miss teaching the most.

I don't want to go back to worrying that what I'm saying isn't important, because it is.

There just seems to be so much wrong with the world, and I feel its pain. I don't know what to do. There is so much I want to change. How can I make those changes? Why do I think the changes need to be made?

I'm not sure if this even makes any sense, as I'm half-crocked on pain meds and wondering why I'm at the computer at all. I think it was to feel something. I've felt numb all day. The movie I just watched, "The Shack," was a very powerful interpretation of what God is, or of how the Father, Son, and Holy Spirit are always with us. Did I doubt this knowledge? Do I believe it? I want to. I want to believe there is good left in the world.

Things seem so different from when I was growing up. Back then, everything seemed to have more meaning and we put more time and effort into our lives. Now we just take everything for granted; we take people and jobs and money and especially our health for granted.

What is the key to happiness? Is it true love, money, property, fame, all of the above?

I've been happy, even though there are times that seem impossible. Weren't we meant to fight for survival? What about those who stand by and watch? Do they learn the same lessons as those of us whom have really suffered? Or is it us that missed the lesson? Who knows? I just want to know it all hasn't been a waste of time. Like today.

~

As I've said before—and as you can see from my journal entries above—I still have my bad days along with my good ones. It's okay to be angry and frustrated about with living with chronic pain and illness; let's be honest, it totally sucks!

There is hope in this story of mine, and there is hope for you as well. Be okay with where you're at now and allow yourself to have a day of rest if needed. Don't judge yourself, and don't allow other people's thoughts into your head. What other people think of you is none of your business. Get out of your own way and let your higher power guide you. Take help when it's offered. Your situation isn't just about you; it presents an opportunity for others to be impacted and blessed by what they can do for you as part of their own growth. It's in our DNA to be nurturing, so don't deny that experience for someone reaching out to you. Cherish and appreciate your true friends and let them be part of this amazing journey we are on.

What did I learn?

Today I'm celebrating that I haven't given up yet! I celebrate all of the activities of daily living that I can complete, even if it is as simple as taking a shower, doing my hair, putting on makeup, walking without a cane, grocery shopping, or going for a walk. I celebrate that I'm still writing this book two years later, and now I have a publisher! My life is not over; instead, my life is taking a new path, even if it's one I never thought I would go on.

This past week has been a battle with anxiety and fear of rejection. If I speak in public about how well I'm doing now, will people believe my story? If I get in shape and start exercising now because I have more mobility, will everyone think I was faking it before? This rollercoaster of emotions is exhausting, but we must allow ourselves the grace we would give others. We MUST forgive ourselves for the guilty feelings of not participating on days when our pain and fatigue is too high. Also, we must not to overdo it on the days we feel really good and expect too much from ourselves.

Celebrate the small stuff and share it with others! People tend to be much more enthusiastic when they hear about our accomplishments than when they listen to us complain about what we can't do.

I celebrate that even after letting go of my beloved nursing career, I still have so much to give. I'm celebrating that I got to use my gifts and make a difference in my own small way. I am neither my illness nor my diseases. I am a useful and much-needed part of my community, with or without my stethoscope.

~

Aug 30, 2017

Recently, a dear friend confided in me about some family and health issues that were becoming overwhelming and how difficult life was for her right then. As I listened, I heard myself in her voice as I have been in her shoes many times. After tearing up a few times, she told me I have been a major inspiration to her and so many others. This couldn't have been better timing for me; my pain levels are better and I'm definitely more mobile, but my weight was at an all-time high. My self-esteem has taken a hit and was chiselling away some of the spunk from my usually chipper self.

I'm just finishing up two months of volunteering for the fires here in BC, where I've been working at the Cloverdale Evacuation site with an amazing organization called the Canadian Disaster Response Team, or CDRT. The fires have been raging for several months now, and with the addition of dry heat and lightning, the Cariboo and Thompson Okanagan are in danger of evacuation. I have over twenty-five years of experience in emergency services, and it was too much for me to just sit at home and watch the situation unfold on TV and do nothing other than to donate cash. Yes, I'm on disability, but that doesn't mean I'm useless: I just have to be careful not to overdo it. I'm a trained experienced professional that's only ten minutes away from the shelter. So, I volunteered with the CDRT for South West BC, which is a non-profit organization that rescues and cares for pets and makes sure their owners have less to worry about during a disaster.

Those who know me are well aware that I don't do anything half assed; it's all or nothing, or at the very least I try to do my best, even if it means putting myself at risk of becoming unhealthy again. This common mistake made by all type-A personalities is a dangerous one, especially for those of us with life-threatening health conditions like systemic lupus. I was forced to retire for one reason: so I could get better. The problem I face, along with many others living with chronic illness, is that my memory seems to favour days where I experience little pain and lots of energy, and I base what I can do on that. Any activity needs to be entered into with caution. I get excited because I'm needed; it makes me feel like I am contributing to the wellbeing of others. I get to use my varied skill sets and show others I'm good at what I do and that I care.

I started working the afternoon shift at the shelter, from 11 a.m. to 3 p.m. Five hours may not seem like a lot to anyone without pain issues, but this is a marathon of a day for me. After two months I was somehow in charge of this site, coordinating staffing and serving as a liaison with the city for new hours and communication with the Regional coordinator. I realize now that I'm still really good, sometimes too good (I always end up in charge somehow); it would have been better to just be a worker bee instead of the Queen. But, I like being the Queen. I like knowing what's going on and helping make our team better and keeping everyone well-informed. So, now that we are near the end our deployment, a veil of sadness and depression covers me. It's over; I'm out of a job again, and I'm no longer needed. The provincial government has deemed that our organization is not needed anymore here in the lower mainland. I realize I have to go back to writing this book, because I know the book is another way I can give back and help people!

This means I have to go back to remembering I'm on disability, and that old familiar grey cloud appears in front of me. I have nothing to look forward to, no lives I can change, and no one to rescue. It's what I know, it's what I do, and it's part of me as a rescuer. I don't know that I'll ever be able to let that go. Enter those five stages of grief—denial, anger, bargaining, depression, and acceptance. I know that we go up and down on this scale and not always in the corresponding order as logic would dictate. It's been twelve years living with chronic pain and illness. It's been two and half years since I had to leave my nursing and education career that I loved. I feel like I have to let go again.

This time, however, I'm grateful that this posting has come to an end for me. I'm grateful to my body for telling me it's time to stop. Grateful to my mind for being gentle in the acceptance of letting this adventure go. And, grateful for the kindness of others that are aware that I need to be done and it's time to take care of me again. I see now that even three days a week for four hours at a time is too much for me. I was coming home exhausted, in pain, agitated, and needing to crash as soon as I got in the door, with nothing left to give my family—much as I did when I was working full time.

I'm grateful for the opportunity to work with amazing volunteers and the new friendships and bonds that have been made. Grateful for my husband that also recognizes I need to rest up now and get better. I'll admit, there was a secret part of me that wondered if I could go back to being a nurse or teaching. I could, but I know I'd be right back where I was two and half years ago. I was unable to walk without the use of a cane and needing to use the handicapped parking spot. I had to ask my family for assistance with simple activities of daily living.

Balance. I need to find balance. I will find balance. I am important. I am needed. Not necessarily professionally, but personally. At home with my family and close friends, where I deserve to be healthy and happy! I am told we may be deployed to another location in Northern BC; I politely decline. Not this time. Not me. It is someone else's turn to shine and my turn to rest. I needed to go through this season, to learn that I can still do a great job of organizing and staying calm in the storm of disaster response. I fear that after completing this book I'll have nothing else to look forward to, no job to be attending, and no more accomplishments to achieve.

There must be more to do. I just need to stop the "what ifs" and keep moving forward. Now that I have that out of my system, I need to go back to my reality of taking care of myself so I can be around longer for my family. I am not quitting, I am not giving up. I'm simply stepping aside so someone else can take their turn.

∼

"There is a time for everything, and a season for every activity under the heavens,"
Ecclesiastes 3:1 (NIV)

Where am I now?

Writing this book was a challenge, but I did it. I look back at the days when it seemed impossible that I could accomplish anything, and I am proud of what I've achieved. In the past three months, I've been hospitalized for a severe kidney infection, then another bladder or kidney infection after Christmas, then a sinus infection that lasted a whole month.

After a two year wait, I was finally accepted into the Pain Clinic and now I'm currently receiving Bilateral Medial Branch Nerve Blocks on my spine. For this procedure, they froze the spinal peripheral nerves for a few hours as a test, making sure that the treatment is effective for me. Next I'll be going for the full cauterization of those same spinal nerve branches in the next few weeks. If this works, I may get three to twelve months of pain relief! This only lasts until the branch nerves grow back, and then they would repeat the cauterization. I'm excited and nervous at the same time. It's quite a safe procedure, but it's extremely painful as you are awake the entire time. This will be a game changer for me and my activity levels, not to mention the positive impact this will have on my self-esteem and on my family.

We've also recently learned that I've been going through menopause as well. So now, on top of everything else, I'm having mood swings, hot flashes, and other annoying body changes; good grief, the Lord has a sense of humour!

Honestly, now that this book is wrapping up, I'm terrified and unsure if I'm ready to release of so much personal information. However, I know in my heart that this self-exposure of pain, illness, and vulnerability will somehow reach out to someone else going through their own challenges, whether it is illness or another personal battle. I found a way to break free from the burden of what I was doing and change my in mindset to be that of "well done." This book may never be a money maker, but it wasn't meant to be in the first place. It was meant to help people understand that they are not alone in this battle. A chronic illness doesn't have to be the end of you. It can't be! Instead, it needs to be your new path. You may not know what that path is or where it will take you, but you must find the courage to continue and follow where it leads. If you fall, you must get back up again, and again, and again, and again, because that's what real courage is; not how much you succeed, but how many times you fall and still continue to get back up each and every time.

My hope for you is that you find some kind of comfort in what I've shared here, or that you can relate to some of my story and feel that you're not alone. Whatever your struggles may be,

I pray that you will be able to reach out to a higher power and receive a loving support system. Your story is important, and your story matters.

We are warriors, we are strong, we are resilient, but most of all, we are not our illness!

"For I know the plans I have for you, declares the Lord, plans to prosper you and not harm you, plans to give you hope and a future."
Jeremiah 29:11 (NIV)

Journal reflection: Have you given yourself the recognition you deserve?

\
\
\
\

Resources

Arthritis Research Canada
Website: www.arthritisresearch.ca
Phone: 1-844-207-0400

BC Lupus Society
Website: www.bclupus.org
Phone: 1-866-585-8787

BC Mobility Opportunities Society
Website:
The College of Family Physicians of Canada
Website: www.cfpc.ca
Phone: 1-800-387-6197

Canada Pension Plan Disability Benefits
Website: www.canada.ca/en/employment-social-development/programs/pension-plan-disability-benefits.html
Phone: 1-800-277-9914

Canadian Association for Suicide Prevention
Website: www.suicideprevention.ca

CDC Canada
Website: www.cdc.gov/globalhealth/countries/canada/

Lupus Canada
Website: www.lupuscanada.org
Phone: 1-800-661-1468

National Benefit Authority—Tax benefits for your disability
Website: www.thenba.ca/disabilities/tax-benefits
Phone: 1-888-389-0080

Pain BC—Connect for Health
Website: www.painbc.ca/chronic-pain/connect-for-health
Phone: 1-844-430-0818

The LifeLine Canada Foundation
Website: www.thelifelinecanda.ca

Author Biography

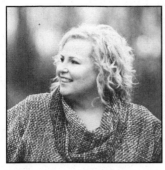

Leisa Cadotte is now retired from her beloved nursing career due to her own serious health complications. Her 20 years' experience in Disaster Response, Search & Rescue, Surgical Nursing and finally as an Educator, allow her to share her expertise and the humor needed to becoming a patient warrior.

Leisa is a passionate and fierce advocate for invisible chronic illness and volunteers with the B.C. Lupus Society and Arthritis Research Canada to raise awareness for these complicated and debilitating diseases such as Systemic Lupus, Fibromyalgia and Osteoarthritis. She also participates as a mentor with multiple online chronic illness and pain platforms. Leisa continues to support health care education and makes guest speaker appearances at the former nursing colleges she used to teach at, as well as sharing her story with other organizations. She is also a true Canadian hockey mom and enjoys watching her son play.

Leisa was born in New Westminster, B.C. Canada in 1969, and grew up in Maple Ridge and White Rock, B.C. She has raised her two boys Mathieu and Benjamin with her husband Francois of twenty seven years, while living in Quebec and Ontario for Francois' RCMP career. They are now back living in Surrey, B.C.

Both Leisa and Francois love the healing properties of the beach and the ocean. You'll often find them with their Goldendoodle Cooper, enjoying the benefits of the salty ocean air and the natural beauty of British Columbia.

More About The Author

Email: leisacadotte@hotmail.com
Website: www.leisacadotte.com
Facebook: www.facebook.com/leisa.k.cadotte
Instagram: www.instagram.com/leisaannking/
LinkedIn: www.linkedin.com/in/leisa-cadotte-1bb12939/